Fundamentals of Emergency Radiology

Fundamentals of Emergency Radiology

Philip W. Wiest, MD

Assistant Professor of Radiology
Veterans Affairs Medical Center
University of New Mexico
Health Sciences Center
Albuquerque, New Mexico

Paul B. Roth, MD, FACEP

Dean of the School of Medicine
Professor of Emergency Medicine
Associate Vice President for Clinical Affairs
University of New Mexico
Health Sciences Center
Albuquerque, New Mexico

W.B. SAUNDERS COMPANY
A Division of Harcourt Brace Company
PHILADELPHIA   LONDON   TORONTO   MONTREAL   SYDNEY   TOKYO

W. B SAUNDERS COMPANY
A Division of Harcourt Brace Company

The Curtis Center
Independence Square West
Philadelphia, Pennsylvania 19106

Library of Congress Cataloging-in-Publication Data
Wiest, Philip W.
    Fundamentals of emergency radiology / Philip W. Wiest, Paul B. Roth--1st ed.
        p.   cm.
    Includes biblioraphical references.
    ISBN 0-7216-5182-8
    1. Diagnosis, Radioscopic.   2. Radiography, Medical.   3. Medical emergencies.
I. Roth, Paul B., 1947– .   II. Title.
    [DNLM: 1. Radiography--methods.   2. Emergency Medical Services.
3. Emergencies.   WN 200 W652f 1996]
RC78.W54   1996
616.07'572--dc20
DNLM/DLC   95-41651

FUNDAMENTALS OF EMERGENCY RADIOLOGY   ISBN 0-7216-5182-8

Printed in the United States of America

Last digit is the print number: 9   8   7   6   5   4   3   2   1

With love to my wife, Anne, and my sons,
Jonathan, Nathaniel, Stephen
PWW

Dedicated to all physicians who are committed
to the reduction of pain and suffering
PBR

Preface

This book is an introduction to emergency radiology for physicians and medical students who will be rotating through an emergency department or urgent-care setting. Our goal in writing this book is to provide a foundation on which these physicians can build experience and expertise in the radiographic evaluation of emergency patients.

Keeping this as a "fundamentals" book has required careful selection of the text and representative images. We have briefly illustrated common illnesses and injuries as well as potential life-threatening problems. The discussions of diseases and trauma are blended with short descriptions of useful imaging modalities. We have also included tables of differential diagnoses and algorithms to help guide physicians through the evaluation of a patient. Each chapter also includes a set of clinical and radiographic "pearls" to help reinforce key concepts.

It is important that physicians who interpret radiographs develop a systematic approach to avoid missing any significant findings. Each chapter has a brief outline on how to evaluate a particular examination that includes a brief differential diagnosis of abnormalities.

We have intentionally avoided referencing the text and instead have provided a list of suggested readings, which includes some of the most complete works written by experts in their fields. This list should prove valuable to those who wish to pursue topics further.

Philip W. Wiest
Paul B. Roth

Acknowledgments

A project of this type requires the assistance of many skilled and talented people. We would like to thank Dr. Fred Mettler, Chairman of the Radiology Department at the University of New Mexico, who provided both inspiration and the resources necessary to complete this project. Members of the University of New Mexico's Department of Radiology who helped review the text include Dr. William Orrison, Dr. Loren Ketai, and Dr. Tom Martin. Jonathan Briggs and his staff, Garbriela Miranda and Percy Bryant, spent many hours typing and editing the text. We are extremely grateful to all of the above for their help. We would also like to express our gratitude to Dr. Michael Davis, the many residents, and Richard Tokarski, P.A., who helped collect many of the images used in this book.

Contents

1

Introduction: Emergency Radiology

Nowhere in medicine is there a greater need for interpreting radiographs quickly and accurately than in the emergency department. Emergency physicians are called upon to read plain films covering the entire spectrum of injuries and conditions affecting patients of all ages. Life-threatening disorders must be quickly recognized and treated appropriately. Consequently, knowledge of numerous imaging modalities is essential to ensure that patients rapidly receive the best test, with the least risk and the lowest cost. Keeping up with the latest procedures and methods requires constant effort. If there is any doubt as to the correct procedure, it is best to consult with a radiologist.

Emergency physicians are responsible for ordering the most appropriate radiographic study while taking into account the risk of exposing patients to ionizing radiation. That is particularly important for women of childbearing age or women who know they are pregnant (Figure 1-1). Table 1-1 has guidelines for evaluating patients who are or who may be pregnant.

Probably the most radiographically challenging patient for the emergency physician is the trauma victim. These patients can have injuries to numerous organ systems and can be clinically unstable. The emergency physician must rapidly assess the patient and carefully orchestrate the total management of the patient, including the imaging workup. Often, consultation with a radiologist is needed to arrange other imaging studies or interventional procedures. A guide to plain-film evaluation of the patient with injuries to multiple systems is included in Algorithm 1-1.

Another challenge to the emergency physician is the pediatric patient. Injuries and diseases often appear differently on radiographs of children than of adults. Child abuse is a serious problem that needs to be recognized quickly so that the child can be safeguarded from further harm.

Intravenous iodinated contrast agents are an important component for additional workup of emergency patients. Contrast agents are used for intravenous urograms and for computed tomography examination of the injured abdomen. It is important to ascertain if the patient has had a prior allergic reaction to any contrast agents, diabetes or heart disease. Also, blood samples used to determine serum blood urea nitrogen (BUN) and creatinine levels should be drawn before any contrast agents are administered to patients with potential renal disease.

In summary, imaging studies are paramount to the evaluation of the ill and traumatized patient; however, there are many pitfalls along the diagnostic pathway. With a thoughtful and careful approach to the radiologic workup, many of these traps can be avoided.

TABLE 1-1   Guidelines for Irradiating the Pregnant or Potentially Pregnant Patient

1. Do not irradiate the abdomen, pelvis, lumbar spine, or hips of a woman in the first trimester of pregnancy, unless it is clearly medically indicated.
2. Whenever possible, defer the examination or choose an alternative imaging modality (for example, ultrasound).
3. Limit the number of images or views obtained to those required to ensure adequate care when evaluating a pregnant woman with modalities that use ionizing radiation.
4. If the abdomen or pelvis of a pregnant patient is accidentally irradiated, the radiology department needs to be notified. The Radiation Safety Officer can estimate the radiation dose to the fetus. This calculation can be used to determine potential effects to the fetus.

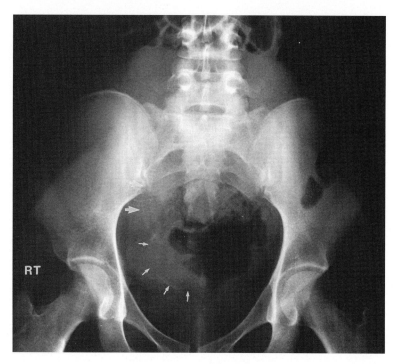

FIGURE 1-1   **AP pelvis: Intrauterine pregnancy:** An AP view of the pelvis of this young female was obtained as part of a trauma protocol after she was involved in a motor vehicle accident. Although the bones are intact, it is obvious that the patient is pregnant. The fetal calvarium is visible in the vertex position (small arrows), and the fetal spine is clearly visible on the right side (large arrows). No consistent scientific evidence indicates that the fetus is harmed at dose levels used in diagnostic radiology. Ionizing radiation is most harmful to the developing fetus during weeks 8 through 16 of gestation when the organs (especially the brain) are developing.

ALGORITHM 1-1   **Plain Film Evaluation of the Multi-System Trauma Patient**

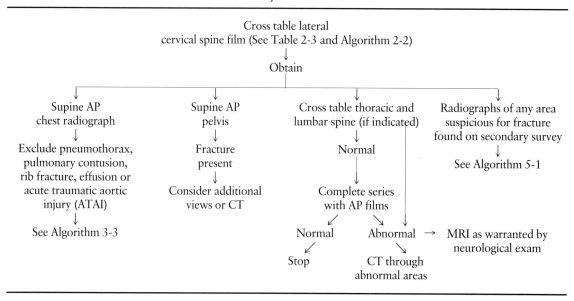

2

Neuroradiology: Head and Spine Evaluation

OVERVIEW

Patients coming to the emergency department with severe headache, first-time seizure, localizing neurologic defects, or head trauma are frequently evaluated using radiographic tests to diagnose their condition.

TECHNIQUES

Plain-Film Radiography

Although "skull films" were the predominant method of evaluating the calvarium in years past,

they have limited usefulness for head trauma evaluation and have been superseded by computed tomography and magnetic resonance imaging. Plain-film radiographs of the skull, however, continue to play an important role in the skeletal survey of a child suspected of being abused.

When evaluating plain films for the possibility of skull fracture, certain diagnostic keys must be considered. Fractures are usually linear in nature (Figure 2-1). Depressed fractures account for only a small portion of bony trauma to the skull and are more commonly seen in children (Figure 2-2). Linear

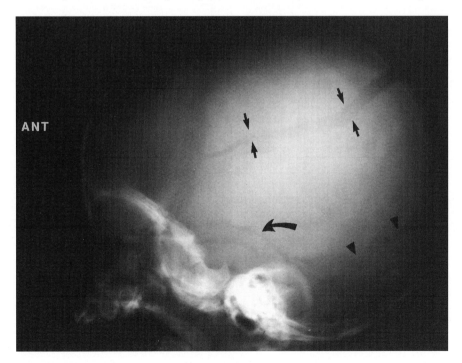

FIGURE 2-1 **Lateral skull: Skull fracture:** This young child has a parietal skull fracture (arrows). Note that the fracture is linear and lacks any branches, two characteristics of skull fractures. Normal cranial sutures are also demonstrated (curved arrow and arrowheads).

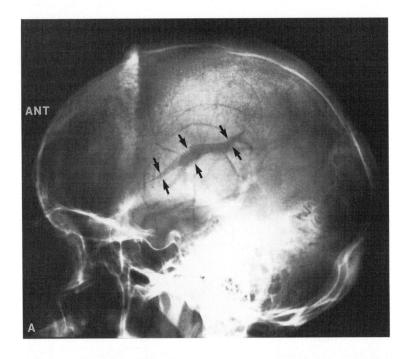

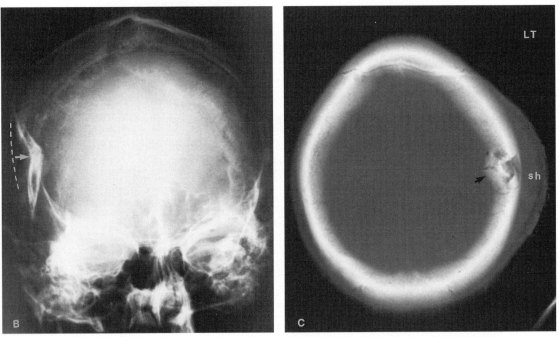

FIGURE 2-2   **Skull plain films and cranial CT: Depressed skull fracture; (2) cases:**   (A) Lateral skull radiograph demonstrates an obvious parietal skull fracture (arrows). The stellate appearance of the fracture suggests a depressed component. (B) The AP view is remarkable for a significant depressed skull fragment (dashed line and arrow). (C) Cranial CT done with bone technique of a different patient reveals a high left parietal depressed skull fracture (arrow). A large scalp hematoma (sh) also is present.

fractures appear as a lucent line that crosses vascular channels and sutures and demonstrates no branching, thereby distinguishing them from either cranial sutures or vascular grooves. Because fractures cross both the inner and outer tables of the skull, they are more lucent than vascular grooves, which are confined to only one table of the skull. Usually cranial sutures only cause diagnostic confusion in the pediatric population because of their unfused appearance. Sutures have a characteristic location and, with the exception of the sagittal suture, are usually bilaterally symmetric. As the child ages, the sutures take on a characteristic serpiginous appearance and eventually fuse.

Computed Tomography (CT)

Computed tomography (CT) is the mainstay of emergent diagnostic neuroradiology. Most CT is performed without intravenous contrast agents because these agents have limited usefulness in the evaluation of acute neurologic abnormalities. Normal enhancement of intracranial structures makes it difficult to exclude subarachnoid hemorrhage or

small extra-axial hemorrhages when using contrast. Furthermore, patients requiring additional workup other than noncontrast cranial CT, are usually evaluated with magnetic resonance imaging (MRI).

CT scans may be normal during the acute phase of many neurologic abnormalities including ischemic infarcts, early infections, and trauma. Follow-up CT or MRI may be necessary for an accurate diagnosis.

It is important to maximize the diagnostic capabilities of CT by obtaining scans at multiple window and level settings. Computer manipulation of these two factors makes it possible to accentuate either bone or soft-tissue detail (Figure 2-3). Table 2-1 outlines the evaluation of noncontrast cranial CT.

Magnetic Resonance Imaging (MRI)

MRI has limited usefulness in evaluating cortical bone. It does, however, provide superior evaluation of soft tissues including brain and spinal cord parenchyma. It is more sensitive than CT in the detection of early parenchymal abnormalities as well as small fluid collections.

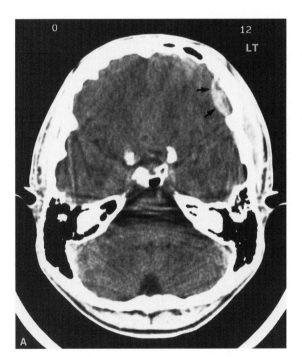
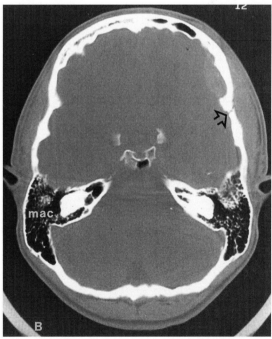

FIGURE 2-3   Noncontrast cranial CT: Epidural hematoma and skull fracture; effect of windows and level settings: Axial CT through the skull base of this trauma patient was done with two different window and level settings. In (A), the image data was manipulated to accentuate the soft tissues. A small left frontal epidural hematoma is visible (arrows). Image (B) is the same slice, but the data was manipulated to enhance bony detail. A nondisplaced temporal bone skull fracture (open arrow) is visible. Changing the window and level settings increases the diagnostic capability of CT. Note the well-pneumatized mastoid air cells (mac). Any opacity of these air cells is pathologic and may indicate infection or a basilar skull fracture.

TABLE 2-1   Evaluation of Cranial CT without Contrast

Structure	Radiographic Finding	Common Differential Diagnosis

Brain Parenchyma	Low attenuation lesions; "Dark area" (but not as dark as CSF)	Cerebral edema from:
		  trauma
		  infarct
		  tumor
		  infection

	High attenuation lesions; "White area"	Acute hemorrhage Intracranial calcification Intracranial foreign bodies, i.e., bullet fragments

	CSF density	Encephalomalacia from prior:
		  trauma
		  infarct
		  surgery

Ventricles	Midline position	Normal

	Off midline	Mass effect from:
		  edema
		  hemorrhage
		  tumor

	Small size to nonvisualization	Cerebral edema (exclude brain herniation)
	Large size	Hydrocephalus Cortical atrophy
Subarachnoid spaces and basilar cisterns	Present and symmetric	Normal
	Effaced or asymmetric	Mass effect Filled with isodense fluid (SDH)
	CSF density	Normal
	High attenuation fluid	Acute blood Inflammatory debris
Cortical sulci	Present and symmetric	Normal
	Effaced	Mass effect Filled with isodense fluid (SDH)
	Large	Cerebral atrophy
Extra-axial fluid	(see Table 2-2)	
Skull	+/− fractures	
Sinuses and mastoid air cells	Opacification	Infection Blood secondary to trauma (exclude basilar skull fracture)
Scalp and soft tissue	Air	Laceration
Other	Pneumocephalus	Fracture through paranasal sinuses Penetrating cranial trauma

NORMAL BRAIN ANATOMY

The cerebral hemispheres are symmetric structures. When a subtle abnormality is seen, it can be helpful to make a comparison with the contralateral hemisphere to gain additional information. X-rays do not penetrate different densities of body tissue equally. This difference in attenuation explains how structures and pathology are displayed on CT scans. Calcification and acute blood have high attenuation characteristics and appear white. Cerebrospinal fluid appears black due to its low attenuation. Soft tissues are in between and are varying shades of gray. Intracranial abnormalities are categorized according to their relationship to the brain. Intra-axial lesions are located within the brain or spinal cord substance. Extra-axial lesions are outside the brain and include the meninges, ventricles, and skull. These categories assist in outlining an appropriate differential diagnosis for abnormal findings. Figure 2-4 demonstrates the appearance of normal brain anatomy on CT.

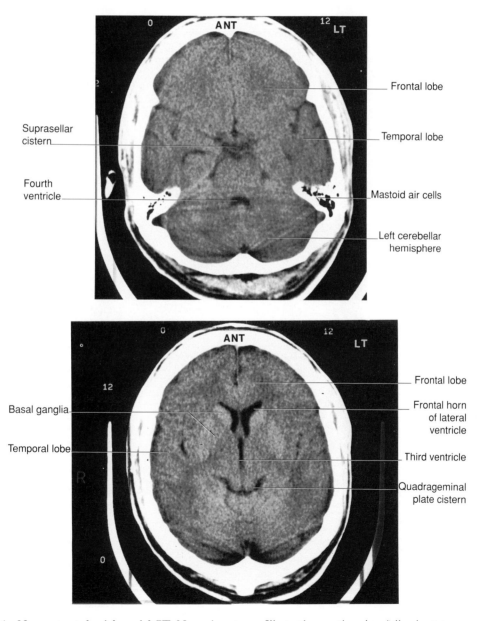

FIGURE 2-4 **Noncontrasted axial cranial CT:** Normal anatomy. *Illustration continued on following page.*

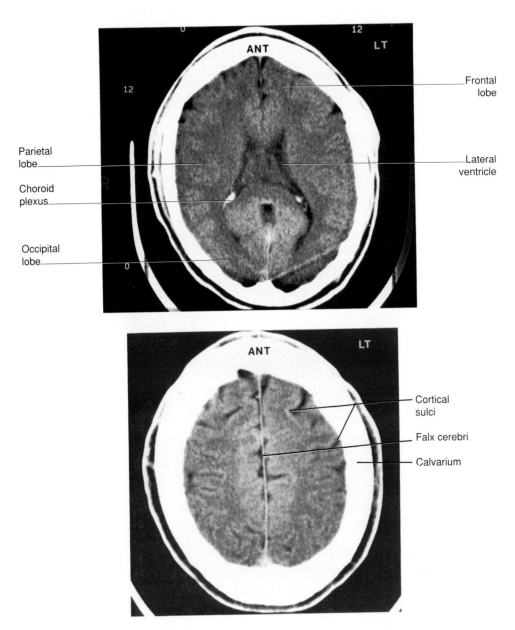

FIGURE 2-4 (continued).

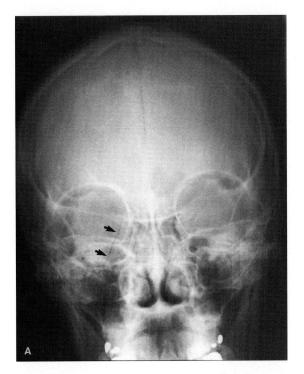 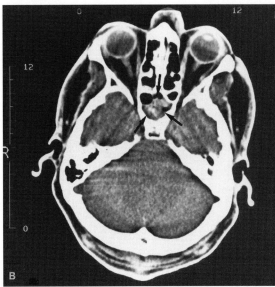

FIGURE 2-5   **Skull plain film and cranial CT: Basilar skull fracture (2) cases:** AP skull film (A) reveals an abnormal lucency through the skull base (arrows) diagnostic of a basilar skull fracture. This was a fortuitous finding as plain skull radiography is not indicated in the evaluation of cranial trauma. In (B), axial CT image through the skull base of a different trauma patient demonstrates two abnormal findings. First, there is opacification of a majority of the sphenoid sinus (arrows). This suggests a basilar skull fracture. Second, another very worrisome finding, is absence of the fourth ventricle. This represents transtentorial herniation from cerebral edema. The patient died a short time after these images were obtained.

SKULL EVALUATION

There is little correlation between calvarial bony injury and underlying brain damage. The primary clinical concern when encountering a patient with cranial trauma is the possibility of an underlying brain injury or extra-axial fluid collection. CT of the brain makes it possible to evaluate not only the soft tissues but also the skull.

Basilar skull fractures are extremely difficult to detect on plain films. Usually there is a significant history of trauma to warrant cranial CT. Sometimes it is possible to detect a lucency through the skull base compatible with a basilar skull fracture (Figure 2-5A); however, often the diagnosis is inferred by detecting fluid in the sphenoid sinus (Figure 2-5B), mastoid air cells, or middle ear. If necessary, additional thin-section CT of the skull base may be diagnostic.

Fractures through the paranasal sinuses, the mastoid air cells, or penetrating cranial trauma can result in intracranial pneumocephalus (Figure 2-6). This is most commonly seen following fracture of the frontal sinus (Figure 2-7). Associated tearing of the dura

may occur and this may be complicated by a persistent CSF (cerebrospinal fluid) leak and meningitis.

Facial Fractures

Plain-film radiographic evaluation of facial injuries is usually reserved for patients with a low likelihood of fracture or for patients with suspected limited fractures such as an isolated zygomatic arch or mandible fracture. Plain films can be useful to screen the trauma patient who is too unstable for CT evaluation.

Facial skeletal anatomy is difficult to interpret in the best of circumstances. Therefore, plain films must be adequate both in technique and in positioning for proper evaluation. Overlying soft-tissue injury as well as nasogastric tubes or endotracheal tubes affect image interpretation. Direct signs of fracture include the obvious cortical break or separation. Other indicators include abnormal linear densities or abnormal cortical angulation. Indirect indicators of facial fracture include soft-tissue

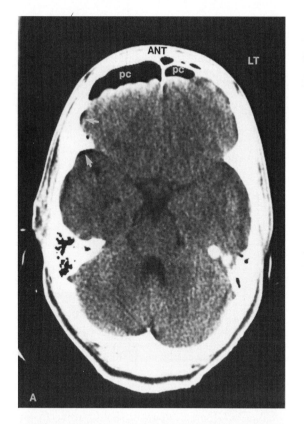

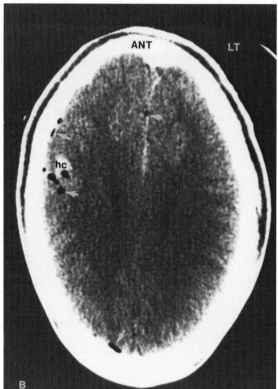

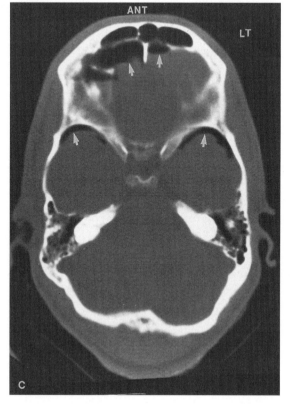

FIGURE 2-6 **Cranial CT: Pneumocephalus:** Axial images (A,B) demonstrate multiple small collections of air (arrows). Extensive pneumocephalus (pc) is present anterior to the frontal lobes. The air is more extensive anteriorly as the patient is supine. A small hemorrhagic contusion (hc) is noted in the right parietal lobe. An axial CT image done with bone technique (C) highlights the intracranial air adjacent to both the frontal and temporal lobes (arrows).

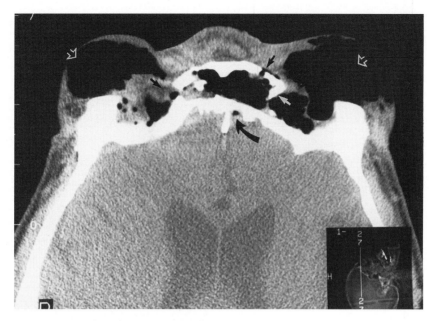

FIGURE 2-7   **Coned-down axial CT frontal sinus: Frontal sinus fracture with pneumocephalus:** There is a comminuted fracture of the frontal sinus with displaced fracture fragments (arrows). A small area of pneumocephalus is present (curved arrow). Bilateral orbital emphysema is visible (open arrows).

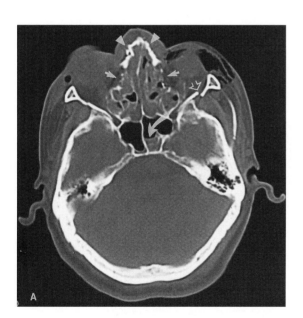

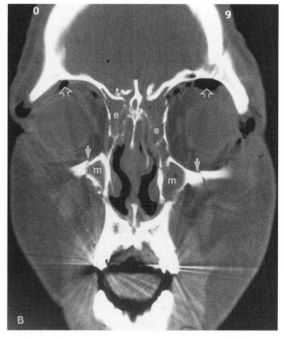

FIGURE 2-8   **Axial and coronal facial CT: Numerous facial fractures:** (A) Axial CT demonstrates numerous fractures including; bilateral medial blowout fractures of the orbits (arrows), fractured nose (arrowheads), left lateral orbital wall (open arrow) and blood in the sphenoid sinus suggesting a basilar skull fracture (curved arrow). (B) Coronal facial CT of the same patient reveals other multiple fractures. Both inferior orbital floors are disrupted (arrows). There is opacification of the maxillary (m) and ethmoid (e) sinuses from blood. Orbital emphysema is present bilaterally (open arrows).

swelling, orbital or subcutaneous emphysema, and opacification of the paranasal sinuses.

High-resolution, thin-section CT is the primary imaging modality to evaluate severe facial trauma. CT is a valuable tool when imaging facial trauma. Small bones and soft tissues are well seen. Computer manipulation of image data allows visualization of facial structures in sagittal and coronal planes (Figure 2-8).

Penetrating eye injuries are a serious threat to the patient's visual acuity. High-velocity missiles, stab wounds, and blunt orbital trauma can cause significant ocular damage that can be difficult to diagnose. Skull and facial radiographs can assist in diagnosing fractures and identifying large metallic foreign bodies but are limited in their ability to detect significant eye injury and small foreign bodies. Thin section CT scanning in the axial and coronal planes is the procedure of choice when radiologic imaging studies are needed to evaluate the orbit and its contents.

Tripod Fracture

Trauma over the malar eminence can result in fracture of the zygoma in three places; the orbital process, the arch, and maxillary process. This is known as a tripod fracture, and it is the most common fracture of the facial skeleton (Figure 2-9). Direct trauma to the zygomatic arch may result in an isolated fracture with a depressed fragment. This is easily overlooked on standard facial films and a bucket-handle view may be necessary to confirm the diagnosis (Figure 2-10).

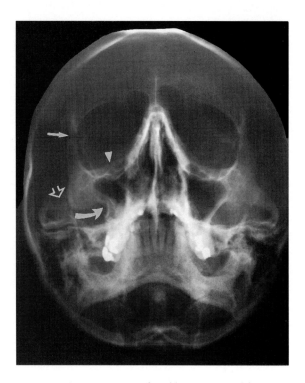

FIGURE 2-9   Waters view facial bones: Tripod fracture: Direct trauma to the malar eminence can fracture the zygoma in three characteristic areas: the lateral orbital wall (arrow); the zygomatic arch (open arrow); and the maxillary process including the inferior rim of the orbit (arrowhead) and the lateral or posterior wall of the maxillary sinus (curved arrow). This fracture complex is commonly known as a tripod fracture. A more appropriate and descriptive term is zygomaticomaxillary fracture.

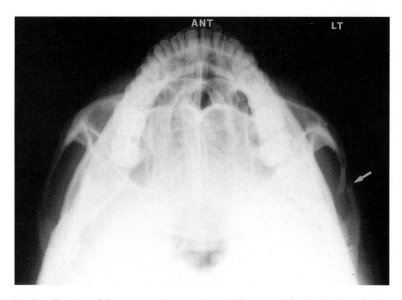

FIGURE 2-10   Bucket-handle view of the zygoma: Zygomatic arch fracture: The bucket-handle view is used specifically to examine the zygomatic arch. A depressed fracture is visible on the left (arrow). The zygomatic arch on the right is normal.

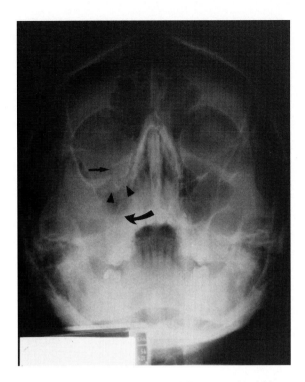

FIGURE 2-11 Waters view facial bones: Orbital blow-out fracture: A fracture through the inferior orbital rim is identified in this patient who was struck in the eye (arrow). A convex mass is seen projecting into the roof of the maxillary sinus representing displaced periorbital tissues (arrowheads). An air-fluid level is present in the maxillary sinus (curved arrow) representing blood.

Orbital floor fractures are commonly seen in association with more complex facial injuries. However, they may be isolated injuries secondary to a direct orbital blow. Classically, the inferior orbital blow-out fracture is manifested by opacification of the maxillary sinus with the appearance of a convex mass projecting into the roof of the maxillary antrum (Figure 2-11). This convex mass represents intraorbital tissues that have been displaced through a fracture in the orbital floor.

Mandible fractures usually occur through the mandibular body, with a high association of multiple fractures in the mandibular arch. Therefore, a search for a second fracture is necessary. An additional fracture is commonly found in the mandibular angle (Figure 2-12). Mandibular fractures are frequently associated with mid-face fractures and may be difficult to detect in the comatose or severely injured patient.

TRAUMATIC BRAIN EMERGENCIES

Significant post-traumatic findings on cranial CT usually center around the identification of areas of abnormal brain attenuation, mass effect, extra-axial fluid collections, or skull fracture.

Cortical Contusions

Cortical contusions present as focal areas of abnormal attenuation indicating injury to brain matter. Such focal areas are commonly seen in the anterior temporal lobe and frontal lobe regions. Contusions tend to be multiple and commonly hemorrhagic in their appearance (Figures 2-13). Non-hemorrhagic cortical contusions are difficult to detect initially and follow-up scans demonstrate developing areas of edema. Contusions occurring directly beneath the area of trauma are known as coup injuries, and damages occurring on the opposite side of the cranial impact are known as contra-coup injuries. A hemorrhagic contusion may be difficult to differentiate from an acute intracerebral hematoma. MRI is more sensitive than CT in detecting cortical contusions and white-matter injury and may be beneficial to obtain in the postconcussive patient with an altered sensorium.

FIGURE 2-12 Panorex view: Fractured mandible: A displaced paramedian fracture of the symphysis (arrows) is visible in association with a fracture through the mandibular angle (curved arrow).

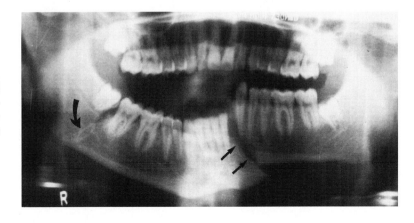

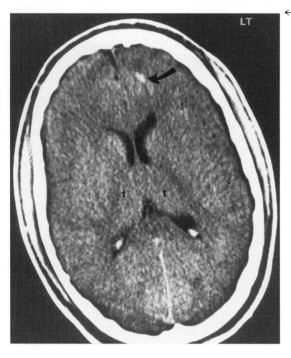

← FIGURE 2-13 **Noncontrast cranial CT: Frontal lobe contusion:** An Axial CT image through the level of the thalamus (t) reveals a small area of increased attenuation in the left frontal lobe (curved arrow). This finding indicates a small hemorrhagic contusion.

Intracerebral Hematoma

Intraparenchymal brain hemorrhage occurs secondary to ruptured blood vessels. Intracerebral hemorrhages are commonly located in the white matter of the temporal and frontal lobes (Figure 2-14). Basal ganglia hemorrhages are also common. Differential diagnosis includes trauma, leaking vascular malformations, ruptured aneurysm, hemorrhagic infarct, and hypertensive hemorrhage. Patients on anticoagulation therapy can also present with acute intracranial bleeds.

Hypertensive hemorrhage is a specific type of intracerebral hemorrhage that is commonly located in the region of the internal capsule and basal ganglia. The putamen is the most common area within the basal ganglia to bleed.

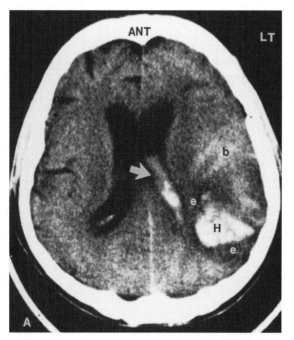
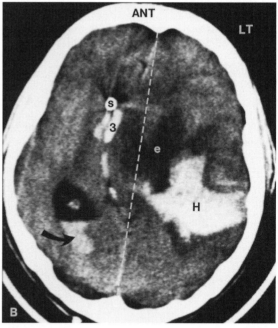

FIGURE 2-14 **Cranial CT: Intracerebral hemorrhage:** Axial CT done at initial presentation (A) revealed a large left-sided posterior parietal hemorrhage (H). Blood (b) is present in the adjacent brain parenchyma. Edema (e) surrounds the large hemorrhage and there is intraventricular expansion of the blood (arrow). Follow-up axial CT (B) was performed after an emergent intraventricular shunt (s) was placed. A dramatic change occurred. The parietal hemorrhage (H) increased in size and the surrounding edema (e) worsened. Both these factors caused severe mass effect with a shift of the midline structures to the right resulting in total effacement of the left lateral ventricle. This indicates subfalcine brain herniation. Blood is present in the third (3) ventricle and there is a CSF-blood level in the posterior horn of the right lateral ventricle (curved arrow). The posterior horn is dilated because the normal CSF flow is obstructed. This represents focal hydrocephalus. The patient died, and a ruptured aneurysm was found at autopsy.

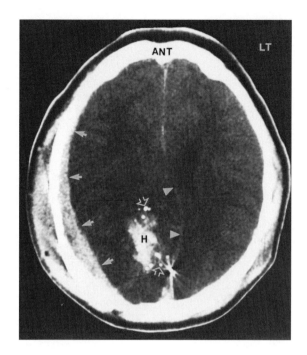

←

FIGURE 2-15 **Cranial CT: Subdural hematoma (SDH):** Axial CT of a gunshot injury to the head reveals numerous intracranial metallic fragments (open arrows). A large parenchymal hematoma (H) and right SDH (arrows) resulted in a right-to-left midline shift (arrowheads). Subdural hematomas have a crescent shape and variable CT attenuation depending on their age and the patient's hematocrit. The high attenuation of this SDH indicates acute blood.

Extra-axial Fluid Collections

The emergency physician must always be alert for a possible subdural or epidural hematoma when examining a patient who has a head injury. Acute extra-axial blood appears dense or white on non-contrast cranial CT. It is classified as subdural (Figure 2-15), epidural (Figure 2-16), subarachnoid (Figure 2-17), or intraventricular (Figure 2-14)

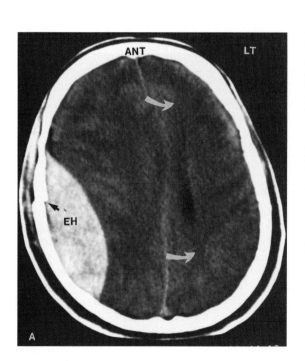

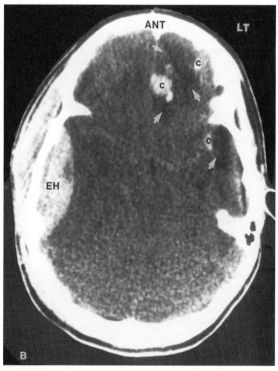

FIGURE 2-16 **Cranial CT: Epidural hematoma (2) cases:** (A) Axial CT of an automobile accident victim demonstrates a large right parietal epidural hematoma (EH). Note the typical biconvex appearance. Epidural hematomas are associated with skull fractures and this image reveals a right parietal bone fracture (arrow). Mass effect and midline shift are present (curved arrows). (B) Axial CT of a different trauma patient demonstrates a right temporal epidural hematoma. Numerous hemorrhagic contusions (c) are present surrounded by low attenuation edema or nonhemorrhagic contusions (arrows).

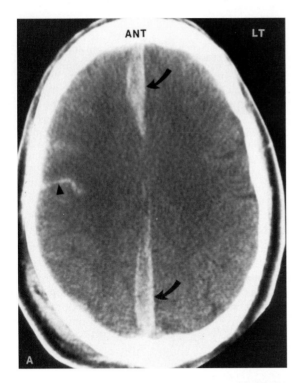

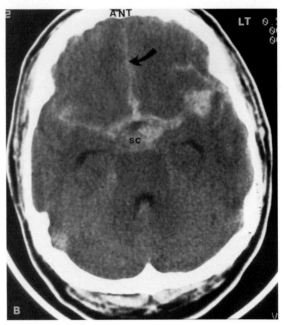

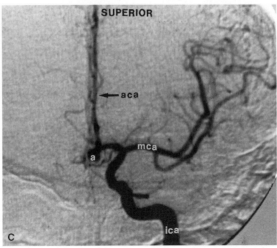

FIGURE 2-17   **Cranial CT and selected internal carotid artery angiogram: Ruptured anterior communicating artery aneurysm and subarachnoid hemorrhage (SAH):** The characteristic finding of a SAH is high attenuation blood located in the basilar cisterns, sylvian fissures, cortical sulci and/or interhemispheric fissure. Axial CT (A) demonstrates blood in both the interhemispheric fissure (curved arrow) and cortical sulci (arrowhead). In (B), blood is visible in the suprasellar cistern (SC). In (C), a selected internal carotid artery (ica) angiogram, an aneurysm (a) of the anterior communicating artery is revealed. The normal anterior cerebral artery (aca) and middle cerebral artery (mca) are also visible. The rupture of this aneurysm caused the large SAH.

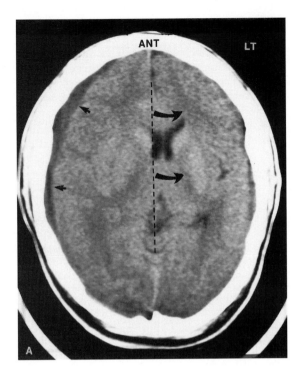
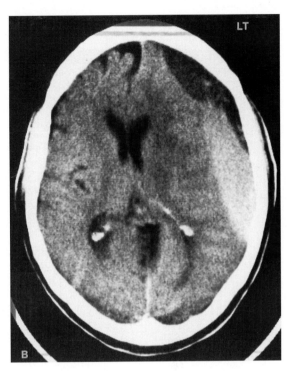

FIGURE 2-18 **Cranial CT: Subdural hematomas (SDH) of varying age (2) cases:** Axial CT (A) demonstrates a low attenuation extra-axial right-sided fluid collection (arrows). This finding is consistent with a chronic SDH. Note the considerable mass effect and midline shift (curved arrows). Axial CT (B) of a different patient shows a large left-sided subdural fluid collection with a fluid-fluid level. The high attenuation component represents more acute blood. This finding is visible in patients with clotting disorders or in patients who actually hemorrhage into a chronic SDH. As in (A), note the corresponding mass effect.

according to its appearance and location. As a subdural hematoma (SDH) ages, it proceeds through a characteristic degradation process with well-known imaging correlates. This is only true, however, in a patient who does not continue to bleed and has a normal hematocrit. A subacute SDH (7 to 21 days) or a SDH in a patient with a low hematocrit can be difficult to diagnose because its CT attenuation characteristics may match the adjacent brain. This isodense SDH may be detected by effacement of the cortical sulci or other evidence of mass effect. When there is doubt, a cranial MRI will be clearly diagnostic. As the SDH continues to age (>3 weeks) it becomes a chronic SDH and becomes less dense than brain on CT (Figure 2-18). Table 2-2 lists the differential diagnoses for extra-axial hemorrhage.

Intracranial Calcification

Numerous normal intracranial structures can calcify. The most commonly seen to do so are the choroid plexus and the pineal gland. Post-traumatic calcification can also occur in the region of prior hemorrhage. However, intracranial processes, both neoplastic and infectious, can present with areas of calcification in either the brain or surrounding structures. Neoplasms that calcify include astrocytomas, craniopharyngiomas, and meningiomas. Intracranial parasitic infections, such as cysticercosis or toxoplasmosis, can also result in areas of dystrophic calcification (Figure 2-19).

Cerebral Edema

Cerebral edema or brain swelling can be a focal or global process. CT demonstrates areas of low attenuation within the brain substance. Edema characteristically has mass effect on adjacent structures. This is manifested by asymmetrically appearing lateral ventricles, obliterated basilar cisterns, effaced cortical sulci, or shift of midline structures (Figure 2-20).

Cranial CT demonstrates a spectrum of findings in cerebral edema from subtle areas of effacement to gross brain herniation. Subfalcine herniation is the most common form and occurs when the cingulate gyrus is displaced across the midline beneath the falx cerebri (Figure 2-14). Another form of herniation is transtentorial herniation of the brain in either a superior or inferior direction across the tentorium. The fourth ventricle becomes effaced with transtentorial herniation (Figure 2-5). Cerebral edema is a finding rather than a disease and can be the sequela of trauma, neoplasm, infarct, or infection.

TABLE 2-2   Differential Diagnosis of Extra-Axial Hemorrhage

Differential Diagnosis	CT Findings	Etiologies	Comments
Subarachnoid Hemorrhage (SAH)	Blood in cortical sulci, fissures and basilar cisterns	Cortical contusions Intracranial hematoma, Ruptured aneurysm, AVM	Blood may block arachnoid granulations and obstruct CSF absorption causing hydrocephalus
Subdural Hematoma (SDH)	Crescent shaped Crosses cranial suture lines but not midline (except in posterior fossa) CT attenuation is variable depending on age of blood and hematocrit: acute blood high attenuation subacute (7–21 days) isodense with brain chronic decreased attenuation resembling CSF	Torn bridging cortical veins	Pay careful attention to subtle mass effect and cortical sulci to detect an isodense SDH Posterior interhemisphere SDH or SDH of varying age in a child is suspicious for abuse Skull fracture uncommon
Epidural Hematoma (EDH)	Biconvex appearance Usually does *not* cross cranial sutures May cross midline	Torn epidural artery- branch of middle meningeal artery Venous bleeding— especially posterior fossa in children	Skull fracture common
Intraventricular Hemorrhage (IVH)	Blood/CSF level layering dependently in ventricles	Torn subependymal vessel Expansion of an intra-parenchymal hematoma	

Hydrocephalus

Hydrocephalus is an increase in the size of the ventricular system, secondary to an obstruction or alteration in CSF flow. The appearance depends on the level of obstruction. Acute hydrocephalus may be manifested by either a focal area of ventricular dilatation secondary to local mass effect (Figure 2-14) or global ventricular enlargement. Traumatic or infectious processes, which subsequently block the ability of the arachnoid granulation to reabsorb CSF, can result in hydrocephalus.

In the pediatric patient, hydrocephalus can result from congenital aqueductal stenosis or other congenital anomalies of brain formation (Figure 2-21).

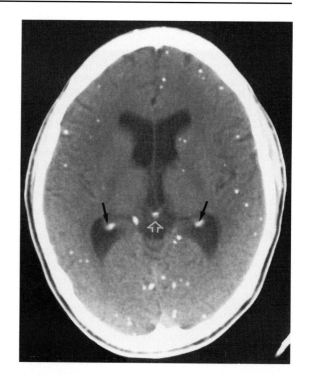

FIGURE 2-19   Cranial CT: Normal and pathologic intracranial calcification: Axial CT shows normal calcification of the pineal gland (open arrow) and choroid plexus (arrows). The remaining scattered calcifications represent the sequelae of chronic neurocysticercosis.

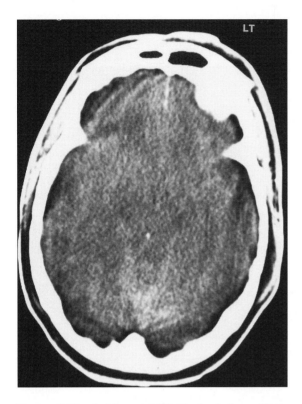

FIGURE 2-20   **Axial cranial CT: Cerebral edema:** Single axial CT image through the brain shows no focal area of abnormal high or low attenuation. This scan is nonetheless markedly abnormal. There is generalized cerebral edema present that has obliterated the basilar cisterns and ventricular system.

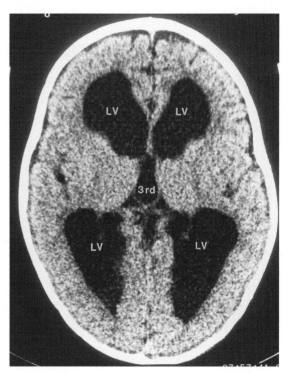

FIGURE 2-21   **Cranial CT: Hydrocephalus:** Axial CT shows marked enlargement of the lateral (LV) and third ventricles. This case of pediatric hydrocephalus was due to aqueductal stenosis.

It is important to exclude mass lesion, hemorrhage, or infection as the cause of the hydrocephalus.

Cerebral atrophy, secondary to progressive loss of brain matter, is common in the elderly. This is manifested by enlarged ventricles with corresponding enlargement of the extra-axial CSF spaces. Prominence of the sylvian fissures and cortical sulci are commonly seen in conjunction with the enlarged ventricles. Findings suggestive of diffuse cerebral atrophy in a young patient are abnormal. Diffuse cerebral atrophy secondary to primary HIV infection is the most common intracranial finding in AIDS patients.

Encephalomalacia

Encephalomalacia is an area of tissue loss. This is manifested on CT by an area of CSF density (dark) in a location where normal brain tissue is expected. Unlike edema, these areas have no corresponding mass effect. In fact, it is possible to identify enlargement of ventricles adjacent to areas of encephalomalacia. This is known as compensatory dilatation. Any process that results in tissue death can ultimately end up as an area of encephalomalacia (Figure 2-22).

NONTRAUMATIC BRAIN EMERGENCIES

Stroke

Stroke or cerebral vascular accident (CVA) is a neurological event categorized by its etiology. The two main categories of stroke are ischemic and hemorrhagic. Ischemic strokes are the most common and can be further subdivided into embolic or thrombotic causes. Embolic disease commonly has a cardiac cause, particularly arrhythmias. Thrombotic causes are secondary to atherosclerotic disease in older patients, and traumatic dissection of the carotid or vertebral arteries in younger individuals.

Many strokes are preceded by transient ischemic attacks (TIAs). TIAs clinically resemble strokes except that their symptoms are transient and last less than 24 hours.

Initial CT diagnosis of an acute ischemic stroke may be difficult because the first CT scan is usually

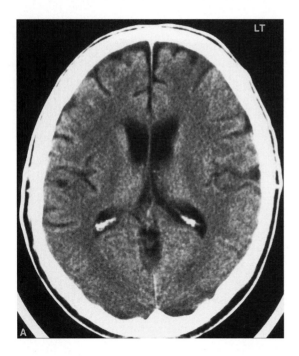

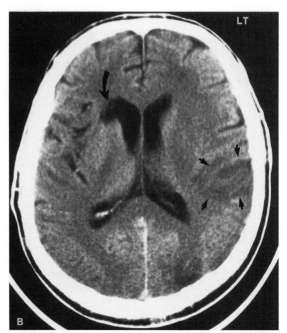

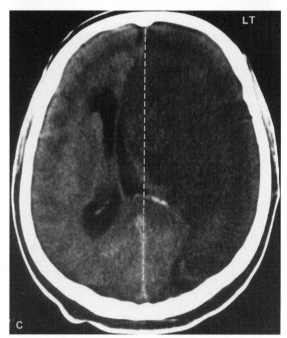

→

FIGURE 2-22 **Axial cranial CT: Evolving infract:** Non-contrast cranial CT (A) shows no abnormality in this patient with a right hemiparesis. Follow-up CT (B) was done 12 hours after admission. An area of edema is developing in the left middle cerebral artery (MCA) distribution (arrows). Also note the small area of encephalomalacia adjacent to the frontal horn of the right lateral ventricle (curved arrow). This area of encephalomalacia represents an old infarct and was present on the initial CT scan, but on a different image than shown here. Follow-up CT (C) 24 hours later demonstrates a massive area of edema involving not only the MCA vascular distribution, but the anterior cerebral artery distribution as well. Note the extensive mass effect on the lateral ventricles and the associated left-to-right midline shift. The patient subsequently died, and autopsy revealed an occluded left internal carotid artery.

normal. However, during the next 24 to 48 hours, CT scans begin to show abnormalities. An area or areas of low attenuation develop corresponding to areas of ischemic or infarcted brain with edema formation (Figure 2-22). These are usually confined to a singular vascular territory and are cortically based. Depending on the severity of the stroke, there can be significant mass effect with shift of midline structures. MRI can detect CVAs earlier, showing areas of abnormal signal in the ischemic areas.

Diagnosis of hemorrhagic stroke is usually made at initial presentation due to the detection of areas of high-attenuation blood. Surrounding low-attenuation edema is commonly found in association with the blood. Like ischemic strokes, severe hemorrhagic strokes may also have mass effect.

Neoplasms

Patients who present with neurological defects, first-time seizures, or severe headaches frequently have CT scans to exclude the possibility of an intra-cranial space-occupying lesion (Algorithm 2-1).

ALGORITHM 2-1 Evaluation of the Adult Patient Presenting with a Severe Headache, Possible Stroke, or First Time Seizure

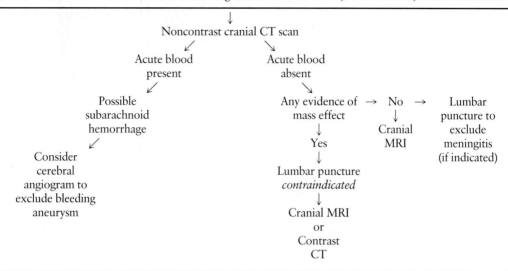

CT appearance of an intracranial mass is usually a low-attenuation lesion with surrounding edema (Figure 2-23). There may be areas of high attenuation associated with the mass, corresponding to hemorrhage or calcification. Melanoma and renal cell metastatic lesions commonly bleed. Again, as with any intracranial process, significant mass effect and midline shift with resultant brain herniation

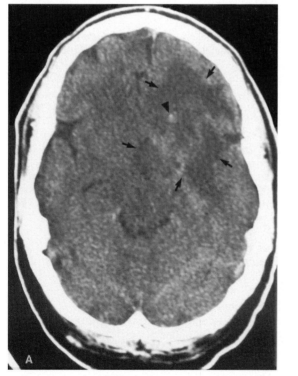

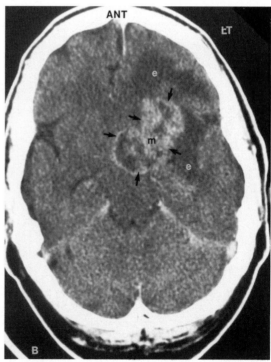

FIGURE 2-23 **Cranial CT with and without contrast: Glioblastoma:** Axial noncontrasted CT (A) shows an ill-defined area of low attenuation in the left frontal and temporal lobes (arrows). A small area of calcification or hemorrhage is visible (arrowhead). Note the asymmetry when compared with the contralateral side. In (B), intravenous contrast has been given and the scan repeated at the same location. A contrast enhancing mass (m) is now apparent (arrows). The surrounding low attenuation indicates edema (e). Biopsy of the mass revealed a glioblastoma.

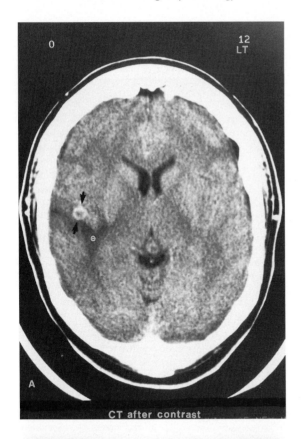

CT after contrast

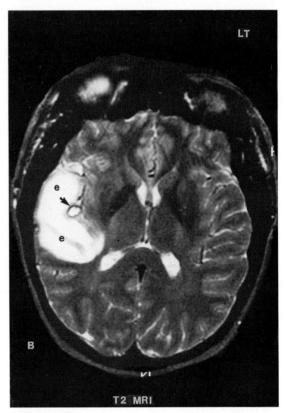

T2 MRI

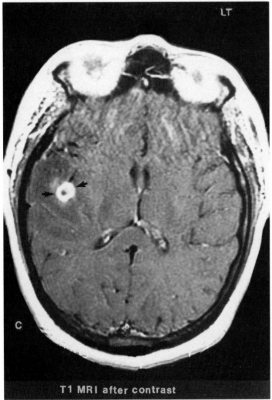

T1 MRI after contrast

←

FIGURE 2-24 **Contrasted cranial CT; pre- and post-contrast cranial MRI: Brain abscess:** Contrast enhanced axial CT (A) shows a small ring-enhancing lesion in the right temporal lobe (arrows). Surrounding edema (e) is present. A cranial T-2 weighted axial MR image (B) reveals a large area of abnormal signal in the right temporal lobe indicating edema (e). Note how much more visible and extensive the edema is on MRI. The ring-enhancing lesion is still visible (arrow). A T-1 weighted axial MR image done with contrast (C) shows the ring-enhancing lesion that was seen in (A). The differential diagnosis of a ring-enhancing lesion includes: abscess, neoplasm, infarct, aneurysm, thrombosed AVM, and resolving hematoma. This was a surgically proven abscess.

may occur. Some tumors are hyperdense when compared with brain parenchyma. Lymphoma, metastatic disease from lung cancer, and melanoma may appear as high-attenuation lesions without associated hemorrhage or calcification.

The differential diagnosis of an intracranial mass depends on the patient's age, location of the tumor (intra- or extra-axial) and history of prior malignancy. In an adult, a metastatic intra-axial lesion is more common than a primary brain tumor.

Differentiation of an intracranial mass lesion from an abscess or infarct may be difficult and depends not only on the history and physical examination of the patient but the patterns of contrast enhancement seen on both CT and MRI. Sometimes, angiography may be necessary.

Intracranial Infection

A brain abscess can result from either direct extension of infection from adjacent structures or hematogenous spread of bacteria. The mastoids and paranasal sinuses are common sites for direct bacterial spread into the cranial vault.

The CT findings of brain abscess depend on the stage of infection. CT scanning of cerebritis or an early abscess may be normal or demonstrate a subtle area of low attenuation. As the abscess matures, necrotic brain tissue becomes hypodense on CT and is surrounded by a "shaggy" capsule that demonstrates enhancement on either contrasted CT or MRI (Figure 2-24).

Meningitis

Patients with headache, nuchal rigidity, and fever are worrisome for having meningitis. The diagnosis is usually made via lumbar puncture; however, pretap cranial CT is commonly obtained to exclude significant mass effect that would make lumbar puncture dangerous. There are numerous etiologies for meningitis including bacterial, fungal, and viral. Noncontrast, cranial CT may demonstrate high attenuation debris in the subarachnoid spaces but is usually normal. Contrasted CT and MRI may demonstrate areas of abnormal meningeal enhancement. Temporal lobe abnormal density and contrast enhancement is characteristic of a herpes-virus meningoencephalitis. Basilar meningeal enhancement can be seen with tuberculosis or other granulomatous causes of meningitis. Hydrocephalus may occur secondary to obstruction of the arachnoid granulations from inflammatory debris.

CERVICAL SPINE EVALUATION

Bony composition of the spine essentially includes the vertebral bodies and the posterior neural arch. Soft-tissue structures responsible for maintaining normal alignment include the anterior longitudinal ligament, the intervertebral disc, posterior longitudinal ligament, and the interspinous ligament.

The most important initial plain film in many traumatized patients is a well-positioned, cross-table lateral view of the cervical spine (Figure 2-25). Appropriate radiographic technique must be used so that all seven cervical vertebra and the C7-T1 relationship is identified. If initial lateral radiographs are unsatisfactory in demonstrating the superior aspect of T1, then special techniques utilizing traction on

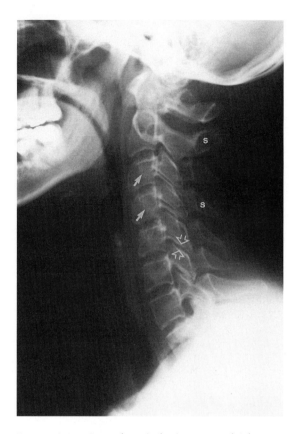

FIGURE 2-25   **Lateral cervical spine: Normal:** This normal lateral cervical spine shows all seven cervical vertebra and the C7-T1 relationship. The vertebral bodies, disc spaces, and alignment are normal. The prevertebral soft tissues demonstrate no abnormal widening. Note the normal cervical lordosis. Other normal findings include: transverse processes (arrows); spinous processes (s); and the superior and inferior facets (open arrows). Refer to Table 2-3 for other normal landmarks.

the arms to lower the shoulders or a swimmer's view may be necessary (Figure 2-26). If these maneuvers are still unsuccessful, then limited CT is indicated. Under no circumstances should the spine precautions be removed unless the lateral cervical spine film is interpreted as normal (Figure 2-27). A normal lateral cervical spine film means that no vertebral body fracture, spine malalignment, or abnormal prevertebral soft tissue swelling is present (Table 2-3).

Normal ranges have been established for maximum soft-tissue width at different levels of the cervical spine for both adult and pediatric populations (Table 2-4). The presence of an endotracheal tube or a nasogastric tube, as well as a film obtained during expiration, can falsely increase retropharyngeal soft-tissue measurements.

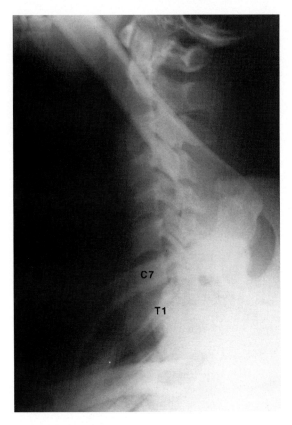

FIGURE 2-26 Swimmer's view cervical spine: Normal: The swimmer's view is a valuable projection to visualize the C7-T1 junction. This view is helpful in evaluating a trauma victim's cervical spine by maneuvering the shoulders out of the way of the cervicothoracic junction.

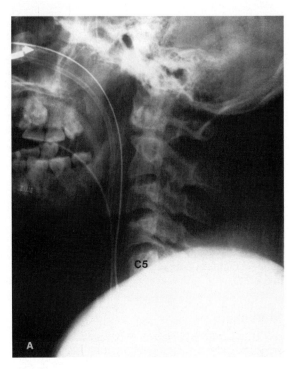

FIGURE 2-27 Lateral cervical spine film, CT and MRI: C6 fracture: This initial lateral cervical spine film (A) of a comatose trauma victim is inadequate because only the top of C5 is visualized. Note the inability to evaluate the prevertebral soft tissues because of the nasogastric and endotracheal tubes. CT through the spine with sagittal image reconstruction

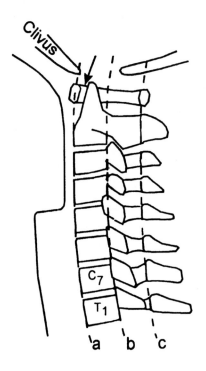

TABLE 2-3   Evaluation of the Cervical Spine "Clearing the C-spine"

1. Examine each spinal line to insure that it is smooth and contiguous. Any interruption is abnormal.
    a. Anterior Spinal line
    b. Posterior Spinal line
    c. Spinolaminal line
2. Examine all seven cervical vertebral bodies to determine the following:
    a. Cortical margins are intact
    b. Height is maintained, no evidence of compression
    c. C7 is in normal alignment with T1
3. Determine whether the spinous processes are intact.
4. Examine disk spaces for abnormal widening or narrowing.
5. Measure predental space (arrow) (see Table 2-4).
6. Examine odontoid process to be sure it is intact and does not protrude into the skull base. The tip of the clivus should point to the tip of the odontoid.
7. Measure prevertebral soft tissues (see Table 2-4).
8. Assess the normal cervical lordosis.

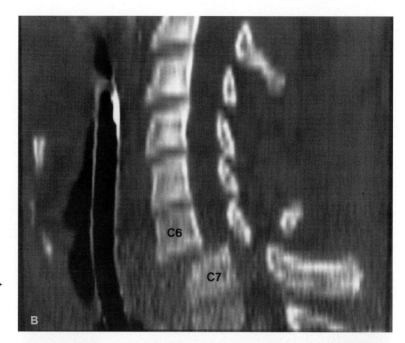

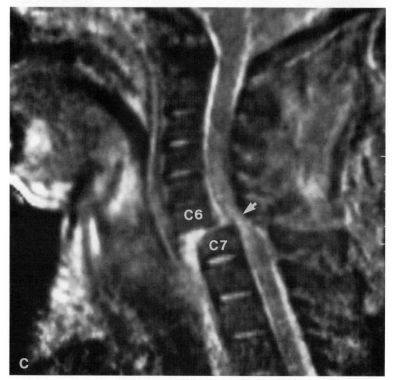

FIGURE 2-27 (continued) (B) clearly shows a fracture dislocation at C6. Sagittal MRI (C) demonstrates C6 anteriorly displaced on C7 and spinal cord compression (arrow). This case clearly illustrates the importance of visualizing all seven cervical bodies as well as the C7-T1 junction on lateral cervical spine films before removing spine precautions.

TABLE 2-4   Normal Cervical Spine Soft Tissue Measurements

Area	Adult	Child
Predental Space	≤ 3mm	≤ 5mm
Retropharyngeal Space Anterior to C3	≤ 7mm	≤ 7mm
Retrotracheal Space Anterior to C6	≤ 22mm	≤ 14mm

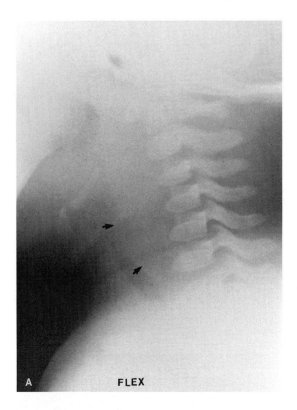
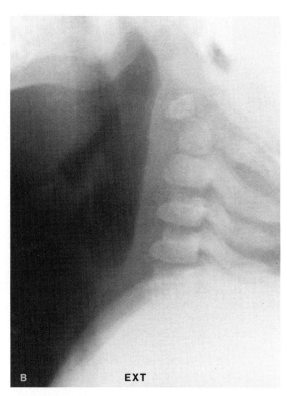

FIGURE 2-28   **Lateral cervical spine: Pediatric flexion artifact:** A lateral cervical spine radiograph obtained with the neck in flexion (A) shows apparent widening of the prevertebral soft tissues (arrows). An additional radiograph with the neck extended (B) demonstrates normal prevertebral soft tissue. This positional variation in soft tissue width is common in children and should not be confused with acute trauma or infection.

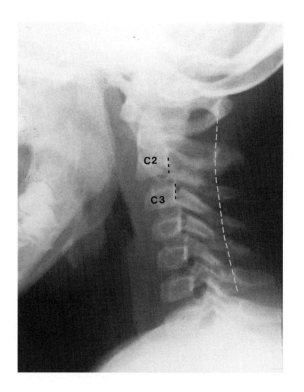

←

FIGURE 2-29   **Lateral cervical spine: Physiologic sublux-ation:** Note that C2 appears to be anteriorly displaced on C3 (black dashed lines). The spinolaminal line (white dashed line) is normal as it intersects the anterior cortex of the spinous process from C1 through C3. This finding is normal in children due to their increased ligamentous laxity.

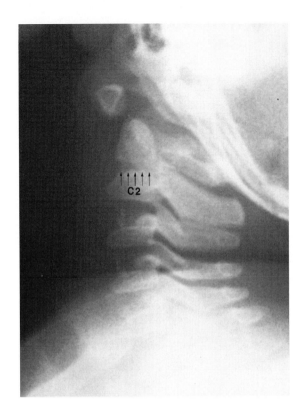

←

→

FIGURE 2-30 Lateral cervical spine: Normal pediatric subdental synchondrosis: The normal developmental subdental synchondrosis is visible as a transverse lucency of C2 (arrows). This should not be confused with a fracture. However, any tilting of the dens or widening of the synchondrosis is abnormal.

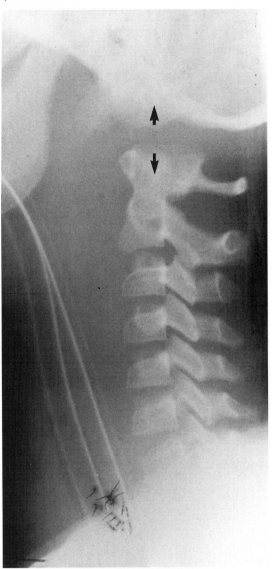

FIGURE 2-31 Lateral cervical spine: Atlanto-occipital dislocation: The atlas (C1) has been dislocated from the skull base (arrows). This dramatic injury can occur from either extension or flexion forces and usually results in sudden death. Note the marked soft tissue swelling in the upper cervical region.

Lateral radiographs of children with the spine in flexion also cause falsely increased soft-tissue measurements (Figure 2-28). Other pediatric considerations include physiologic subluxation of C2 on C3 (Figure 2-29). Due to normal ligamentous laxity of the longitudinal ligaments, the C2 vertebra may show slight anterior subluxation on the C3 vertebra. The spinolaminal line is normal, which excludes traumatic subluxation. The normal subdental synchondrosis is seen as a transverse lucency in the mid portion of the C2 vertebra in children (Figure 2-30). This synchondrosis gradually fuses with age and should not be mistaken for a C2 vertebral fracture. Be careful to inspect this synchondrosis for abnormal widening or tilting of the dens as fractures are common through this area. Fractures of C1 and atlantoaxial dislocations are other less-common pediatric cervical spine injuries (Figure 2-31).

After determining that the lateral cervical spine radiograph is normal, the remainder of the examination should include an AP view, open-mouth odontoid view, and possibly oblique views. The normal AP view should demonstrate spinous processes

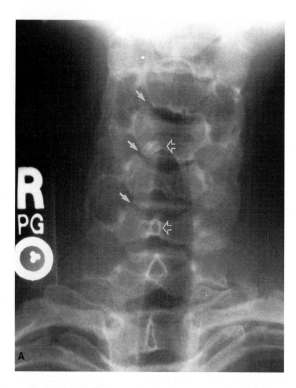

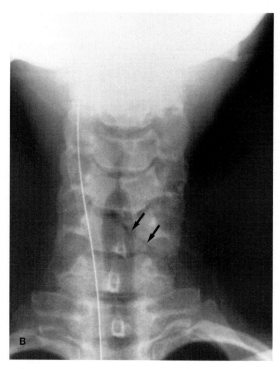

FIGURE 2-32   AP Cervical Spine: Normal and C6 fracture (two cases): (A) AP view of a normal spine shows smooth lateral margins and midline spinous processes (open arrows). The uncovertebral joints are evaluated in this projection (arrows). (B) AP view of a trauma patient who had a normal lateral cervical spine film shows a fracture of the C6 vertebral body (arrows).

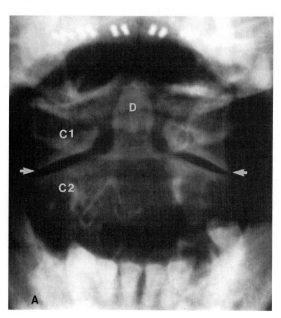

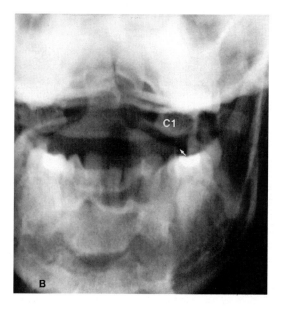

FIGURE 2-33   Open-mouth odontoid view: Normal and C1 fracture (two cases): (A) Note that the lateral masses of C1 are appropriately aligned with C2 (arrows). Any step-off is abnormal and may represent a fracture through the C1 ring. The dens (D) is well seen and normal. (B) Lateral mass of C1 is displaced laterally past C2 (arrow). This is abnormal and represents a fracture of C1.

in the midline (Figure 2-32). Bifid spinous processes are a normal variant. Lateral cortical margins are smoothly undulating. The open-mouth odontoid view evaluates the C1, C2 articulation. Lateral masses of C1 should align themselves with the lateral masses of C2 (Figure 2-33). The odontoid should be intact. The normal gap between the upper maxillary incisors should not be mistaken for an odontoid fracture (Figure 2-34).

Oblique views evaluate the neural foramina, the facet joints, and pedicles. The normal laminae should have a shingle-like alignment (Figure 2-35). Flexion-extension views are obtained to detect soft-tissue injuries. However, acute flexion-extension views are rarely indicated since muscle spasm frequently prevents movement when an unstable ligamentous injury is present. Delayed flexion-extension views (10 to 14 days after injury) will be required to exclude significant injury. On a neutral lateral spine radiograph, vertebral alignment may appear normal. However, with movement, abnormalities in alignment may occur, indicating ligamentous damage. If

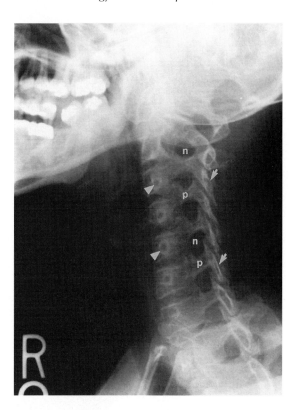

FIGURE 2-35 **Oblique view cervical spine: Normal:** Oblique view is obtained to visualize the pedicles (p), neural foramina (n), and the laminae (arrows). The rounded densities projecting through the vertebral bodies represent the contralateral pedicles (arrowheads).

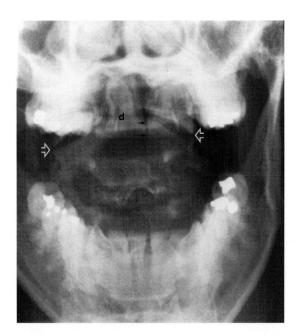

FIGURE 2-34 **Open-mouth odontoid: Artifact simulating fracture:** There is a vertical lucency (arrows) projecting at the base of the dens (d). Closer inspection revealed this to be an artifact caused by the gap between the upper maxillary incisors. The lateral masses of C1 and C2 are normally aligned (open arrows).

flexion-extension views are indicated, patients must perform the flexion and extension maneuvers without any assistance when moving their head. The examination must be immediately discontinued if pain or neurologic symptoms occur (Figure 2-36).

MRI is highly sensitive in the detection of ligamentous injuries and is preferable to flexion-extension views in the acute setting.

Loss of the normal cervical lordosis has been implicated as indicating possible ligamentous damage or cervical muscle spasm. Loss of the normal cervical lordosis can also be an imaging artifact caused by the position of the patient's head. Therefore, when there is clinical suspicion for soft-tissue damage or ligamentous injury based solely on the loss of normal cervical lordosis, obtaining a repeat lateral upright cervical spine radiograph with the head in neutral position or performing an MRI to evaluate the soft tissues may exclude or confirm a diagnosis of ligamentous injury. Algorithm 2-2 outlines the imaging evaluation of patients with suspected cervical spine injury.

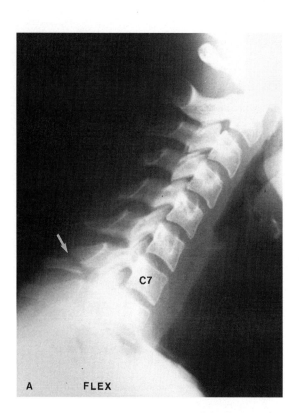
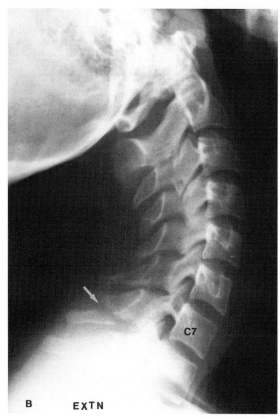

A   **FLEX**   **B**   **EXTN**

FIGURE 2-36 **Flexion-extension views cervical spine: "Clay shoveler's" fracture:** The C7 spinous process is fractured (arrow). This injury is commonly referred to as a "clay shoveler's" fracture as it is seen after strenuous lifting, i.e., shoveling heavy clay. This fracture is also common at C6 and T1. The flexion-extension views are obtained to exclude ligamentous injury. Flexion (A) as well as extension (B) views show normal spinal alignment and no evidence of instability. Flexion-extension views in the acute setting are controversial (see text).

ALGORITHM 2-2   Evaluation of the Patient with a Suspected Cervical Spine Injury

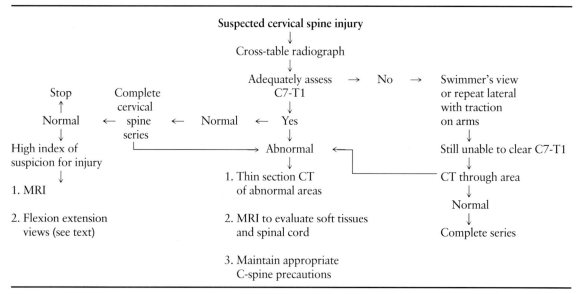

Suspected cervical spine injury
↓
Cross-table radiograph
↓
Adequately assess → No → Swimmer's view
C7-T1   or repeat lateral
↓   with traction
Yes   on arms
↓   ↓
Abnormal ←   Still unable to clear C7-T1

Stop
↑
Normal   Complete
↓   cervical
High index of   spine ← Normal ←
suspicion for injury   series
↓
1. MRI

2. Flexion extension
   views (see text)

1. Thin section CT   CT through area
   of abnormal areas   ↓
                              Normal
2. MRI to evaluate soft tissues   ↓
   and spinal cord   Complete series

3. Maintain appropriate
   C-spine precautions

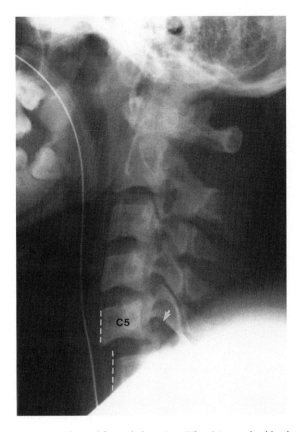

FIGURE 2-37   **Lateral cervical spine: Unilateral facet dislocation:** The C5 vertebral body is anteriorly displaced on C6 (dashed lines). Note the widened and "perched" appearance of the involved facets (arrow) characteristic of facet dislocation.

Various types of injuries have characteristic associated fractures. Flexion forces are the most common cause of cervical spine trauma. Common flexion injuries include anterior subluxation, facet dislocation (Figure 2-37), wedge compression fractures, flexion teardrop injuries (Figure 2-38), and clay shoveler's fractures (Figure 2-36). Compression forces due to axial loading result in fractures of the C1 vertebra and burst fractures of the vertebral bodies. Extension injuries can result in extension teardrop fractures (Figure 2-39), hangman's fractures (also known as a traumatic spondylolisthesis of the C2 vertebra) (Figure 2-40), as well as hyperextension dislocations. Rotational forces can be present with either flexion or extension forces.

Odontoid and dens fractures are classified according to their location. Fractures of the base of the odontoid and the body of the C2 vertebra are the most common. Dens fractures may be difficult to identify on lateral cervical spine films because of overlying bony structures. Abnormal soft-tissue widening may be the only clue indicating a fracture. CT done with sagittal and coronal reconstruction is valuable for evaluating patients with a suspected dens fracture (Figure 2-41).

Additional modalities to assess the cervical spine include CT, MRI, and conventional tomography.

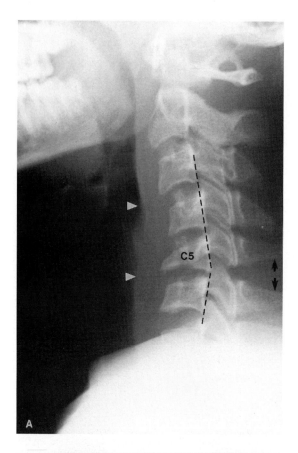

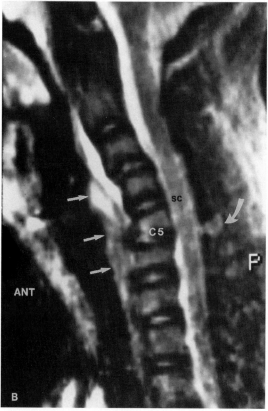

←

FIGURE 2-38 Lateral cervical spine and sagittal MRI: Flexion tear drop fracture: Lateral cervical spine film (A) shows a C5 vertebral body fracture. There is an associated abnormal posterior spinal line (dashed line) and marked prevertebral soft tissue swelling (arrowheads). Abnormal spinous process widening (arrows) represents ligamentous damage from the flexion forces. Sagittal MRI (B) demonstrates abnormal signal anterior to the known C5 fracture (arrows) indicating soft tissue injury. A second, posterior, area of abnormal signal (curved arrow) posteriorly indicates damaged interspinous ligaments. The spinal cord (sc) is easy to see and appears intact.

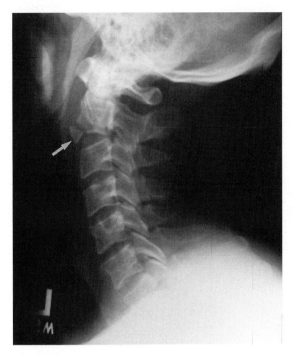

FIGURE 2-39 Lateral cervical spine: Extension teardrop fracture: There is a fracture of the anterior inferior cortical margin of C2. This is secondary to hyperextension forces and avulsion of the anterior longitudinal ligament. This injury is common in osteoporotic patients.

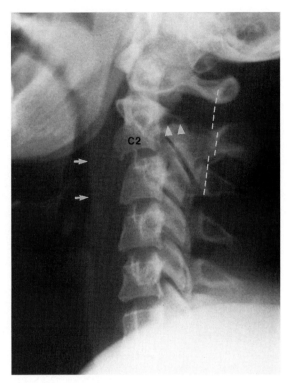

FIGURE 2-40 Lateral cervical spine: Hangman's fracture: A Hangman's fracture goes through the neural arch of C2 (arrowheads) with anterior subluxation of C2 on C3. The spinolaminal line (dashed line) is disrupted and there is soft-tissue swelling (arrows). The name is derived from its similarity to the injury seen with judicial hanging. Hangman's fractures are also known as a C2 traumatic spondylolisthesis and are most commonly seen following motor vehicle accidents with hyperextension forces.

Computed Tomography

CT is advantageous because the patient can be examined while the cervical spine remains immobilized. CT also can be used to further assess areas of suspected injury or characterize known injuries detected on cervical spine radiographs. This additional imaging is beneficial because it provides detail about bony structures and makes it possible to assess the integrity of the spinal canal. Sagittal and coronal image reconstructions, which not only aid in diagnosis but preoperative planning, can be performed. Fractures that appear stable on plain films may be recategorized as unstable fractures once they are better characterized with CT. A disadvantage of CT is that it requires moving the patient out of the controlled environment of the emergency department. Additionally, because of the length of time involved in acquiring conventional CT images, scanning is usually confined to areas of suspected injury. Newer spiral CT scanners can rapidly acquire multiple images and are changing the protocol radiology departments use to evaluate patients with suspected cervical spine trauma.

Magnetic Resonance Imaging

MRI has the advantage in that a larger field of view can be obtained and multiplanar images are a standard protocol of the examination. While MRI is poor at imaging cortical bone, it is superior for evaluating adjacent soft tissues and the spinal cord (Figure 2-27). Disadvantages of MRI include the difficulty in imaging patients who are critically ill or on life support. Other disadvantages include prolonged imaging time and the inability to scan patients with implanted pacemakers and certain other surgical devices such as brain aneurysm clips.

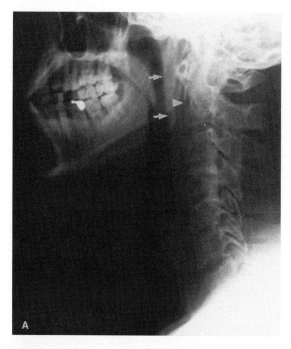

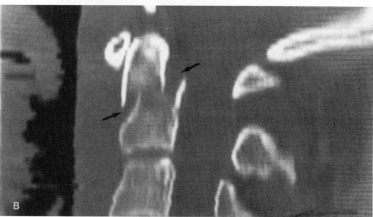

FIGURE 2-41 **Lateral cervical spine and CT: Odontoid fracture:** Lateral cervical spine radiograph (A) shows soft tissue swelling anterior to the upper cervical spine (arrows). There is cortical disruption at the base of the dens (arrowhead). Sagittal CT reformation (B) clearly demonstrates the fracture (arrows).

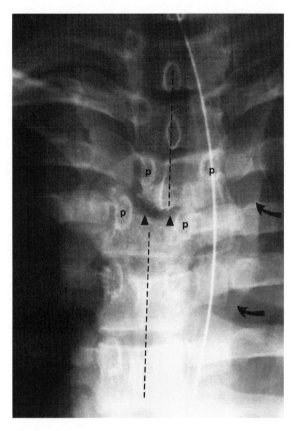

FIGURE 2-42   **AP detail view of the upper thoracic spine: Fracture:** Numerous indicators of fracture are visible on this detail view. The spinous processes (dashed line) and pedicles (p) are abnormally aligned at the site of the fracture (arrowheads). There is a paraspinous mass (curved arrows) centered at the fracture site indicating a hematoma.

THORACIC SPINE EVALUATION

The routine thoracic spine evaluation includes AP and lateral radiographs. These radiographs are used to assure that vertebral body alignment is normal and that the cortical margins are intact. Evaluation of the paraspinous soft tissues is important to exclude the possibility of a paraspinal hematoma or mass. The paraspinous line should be approximately one-third the width of the descending thoracic aorta (Figure 2-42).

Traumatic injuries of the thoracic spine are commonly seen in the thoracolumbar (T11-L4) region. It is common to have multiple contiguous fractures. Vertebral body fractures are commonly wedge- or burst-type injuries secondary to hyperextension and compressive forces. CT aids in the evaluation of any known or suspected bony injury and is especially valuable in the detection of any bony fragments ret- ropulsed into the spinal canal (Figure 2-43). MRI is used to evaluate the thoracic spinal cord as well as the intervertebral discs and paraspinous tissues.

LUMBAR SPINE EVALUATION

Standard evaluation of the lumbar spine is performed in AP and lateral views. Detection of lumbar injury depends on spinal alignment as well as configuration of the vertebral bodies, disc spaces, and spinous and transverse processes. Assessment of the soft tissues for a potential spinal injury is also important, and an abdominal ileus should raise suspicions. Additional views that may be obtained include oblique views to evaluate the pars interarticularis, pedicles, and facets. Oblique views of the posterior lumbar elements in a normal patient form the figure of a Scotty dog (Figure 2-44).

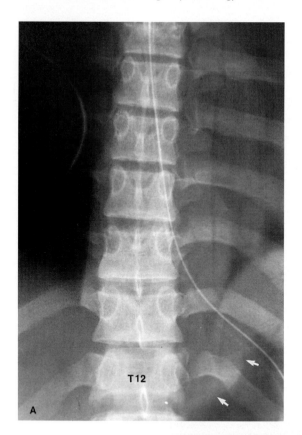

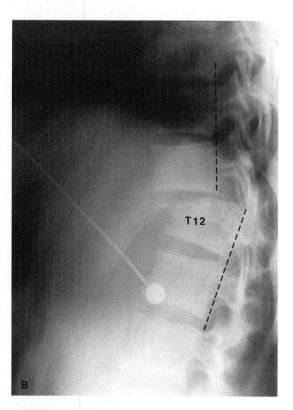

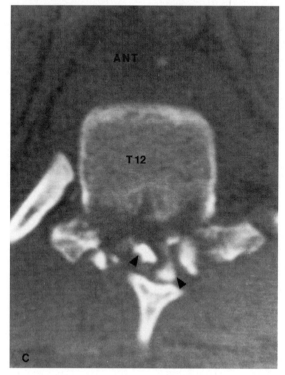

FIGURE 2-43   **AP, lateral thoracic spine with CT and MRI: T12 fracture:** AP view (A) shows a nasogastric tube in the esophogus and stomach. The T11–12 disc space is narrowed and a paraspinous mass is evident (arrows). The lateral view (B) is clearly abnormal, revealing a fracture dislocation centered at T11–12. Note the disrupted posterior spinal line (dashed line) with posterior displacement of T12. Axial CT (C) demonstrates numerous fracture fragments in the spinal canal (arrowheads).

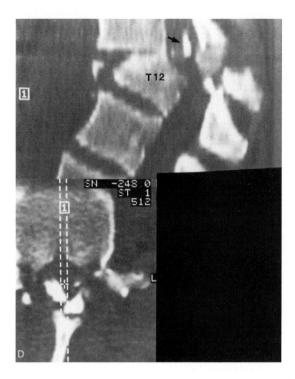
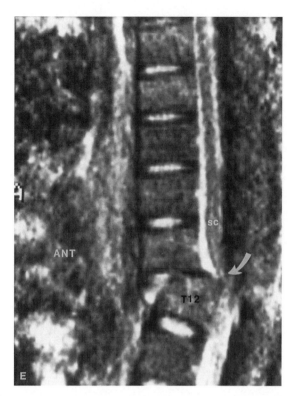

FIGURE 2-43 *(continued)* Sagittal CT reconstruction (D) shows the displaced fragments (arrow) seen on the axial view. Sagittal MR image (E) is remarkable for bony impingement on the distal spinal cord (sc) (curved arrow).

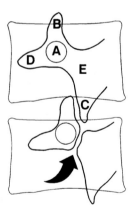

FIGURE 2-44 Oblique view lumbar spine: Normal anatomy and spondylolysis (arrow). A = pedicle; B = superior facet; C = inferior facet; D = transverse process; E = pars interarticularis.

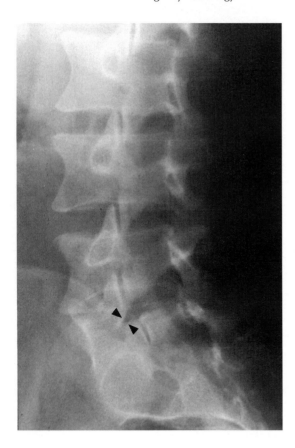

←

FIGURE 2-45 **Oblique view lumbar spine: L5 spondylolysis:** Spondylolysis is identified by the defect in the pars interarticularis (arrowheads).

→

FIGURE 2-46 **Lateral view lumbar spine: Bilateral L5 spondylolysis and Grade 1 spondylolisthesis:** The characteristic appearance of a bilateral spondylolysis on lateral projection is seen at L5 (arrows). There is an associated Grade 1 spondylolisthesis of L5 on S1 (dashed line and open arrow).

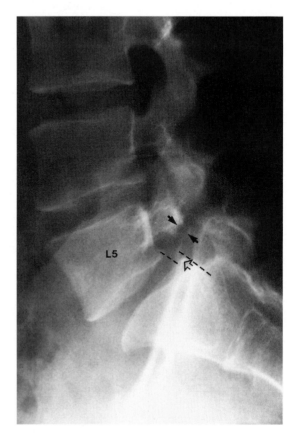

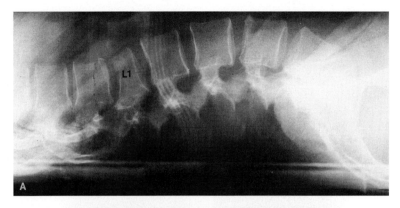

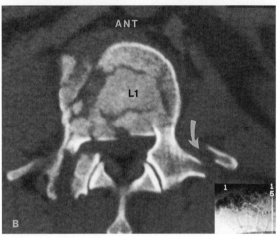

FIGURE 2-47 **Lateral lumbar spine with CT: L1 fracture:** Lateral lumbar spine projection (A) obtained in the trauma room of this accident victim shows a L1 compression fracture. Axial CT (B) reveals the fractured superior L1 end plate. The spinal canal is intact. A transverse process fracture is also seen (curved arrow).

Spondylolysis is a defect in the pars interarticularis (Figure 2-45). It is debatable whether spondylolytic defects are predominantly congenital or post-traumatic findings. Spondylolisthesis is the displacement of one vertebral body in relationship to the normal vertebral alignment. A spondylolisthesis can be asymptomatic or result in significant neuroforaminal stenosis with nerve impingement. Spondylolisthesis is graded according to the degree of anterior subluxation. For example, a Grade 1 spondylolisthesis is offset anteriorly less than 25% of the total width of the adjacent vertebral body. Likewise, a Grade 2 spondylolisthesis is offset less than 50% of the width of the adjacent vertebral body. This classification continues up to Grade 4 (Figure 2-46).

Compression fractures of the lumbar spine are common (Figure 2-47). A less-common fracture of the lumbar spine is a chance fracture. Chance fractures result from hyperflexion forces, causing a distraction fracture through the vertebral body and posterior elements (Figure 2-48). These patients usually are seen after automobile accidents that involved wearing a seat belt without a shoulder harness.

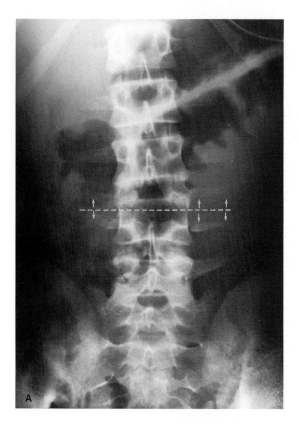
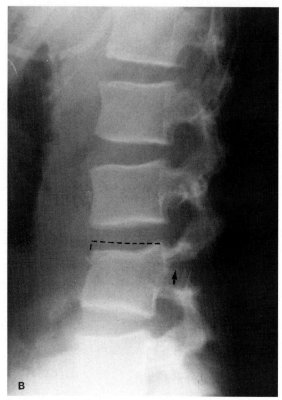

FIGURE 2-48 **AP and lateral lumbar spine: Chance fracture:** The Chance fracture is an uncommon but radiographically remarkable injury of the lumbar spine. Hyperflexion forces result in a fracture through the pedicle, lamina, and spinous process. The AP view (A) shows a fracture plane through L4 (dashed line) that has split the transverse process in half (arrows). Lateral view (B) demonstrates the posterior fracture line through the pedicles (arrow). There is associated wedging of the vertebral body (dashed line).

PATHOLOGIC FRACTURES OF THE SPINE

Pathologic fractures of the spine usually are the result of metastatic disease or osteoporosis (Figure 2-49). It is sometimes difficult to distinguish insufficiency fractures seen in osteoporosis from other pathologic fractures. An adjacent soft-tissue mass suggests a tumor and a metastatic process. However, a paraspinous mass may indicate the presence of a hematoma from an acute insufficiency fracture. Determining the etiology of a pathologic fracture by plain film is difficult, and CT, MRI, or radionuclide bone scintigraphy may be necessary to further characterize it.

DEGENERATIVE DISEASES OF THE SPINE

Loss of the disc space with osteophyte formation can be seen as the patient ages or may represent the sequelae of prior trauma. Hypertrophic changes are common in the spine, usually located in the mid- and lower-disc levels of the cervical and lumbar spine. Alterations in alignment can occur with these hypertrophic changes, and it can be difficult at times to exclude acute bony injury superimposed on chronic degenerative disease (Figure 2-50). In these instances, it is important to remain suspicious until additional imaging modalities, such as MRI and CT, clarify the situation.

→

FIGURE 2-49 **Lateral thoracic spine: Pathologic fracture:** There is a pathologic wedge compression fracture (fx) of T7. Note the increased density of the vertebral bodies secondary to extensive metastatic prostate cancer.

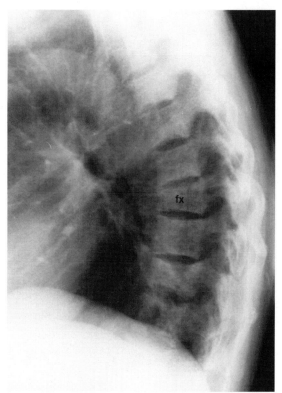

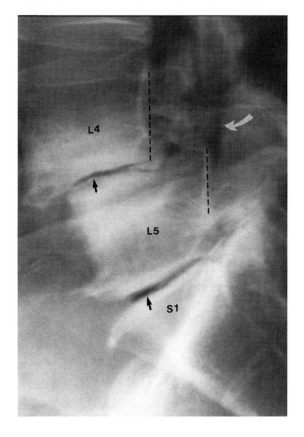

←

FIGURE 2-50 **Spot lateral view lower lumbar spine: Degenerative disc disease:** The L4-5 and L5-S1 disc levels are markedly narrowed with vacuum discs (arrows) present at each level. The vertebral body end plates are sclerotic indicating a chronic process. The L4 vertebral body is subluxed anteriorly on L5 (dashed lines), probably due to a bilateral L4 spondylolysis (curved arrow). Oblique views would be helpful for confirmation. This is a case of long-standing degenerative disc disease. It would be difficult to exclude superimposed acute disease. Prior films, CT or MRI, may be required in the setting of trauma to complete the evaluation.

OSTEOMYELITIS AND DISCITIS OF THE SPINE

Infection of the vertebral bodies and disc spaces can occur at any age. Multiple organisms can hematogenously seed the vertebral body. Pyogenic infections usually cause severe back pain unrelieved by changes in position. Plain-film findings depend on the stage of infection. Early in the course of the disease, subtle disc-space narrowing may be the only finding. As the disease progresses, there is obliteration of the intervertebral disc space and destruction of the adjacent vertebral body end plates (Figure

2-51A). Soft-tissue extension of the infection or edema may be evident on plain film by a paraspinous mass. If untreated, the infection can result in an epidural abscess. Tuberculous or fungal spinal infections present with a more indolent course. Patients at risk for these nonpyogenic infections are the immunosuppressed, including the HIV infected.

CT is helpful in evaluating the bony destruction seen with spine infections (Figure 2-51B). MRI with contrast, however, is the imaging modality of choice because of its superior bone marrow, spinal cord, and soft-tissue imaging.

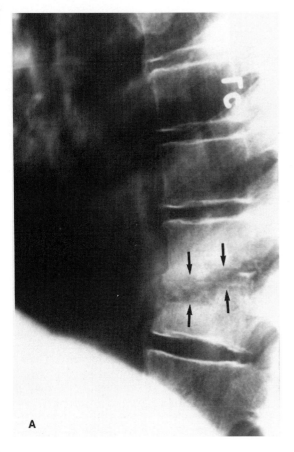

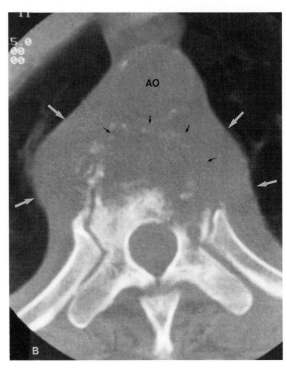

FIGURE 2-51 **Lateral thoracic spine with CT: Spinal osteomyelitis and discitis:** The lateral view (A) shows an obliterated thoracic disc space with destruction of the adjacent vertebral bodies (arrows). Axial CT (B) demonstrates the extent of the destructive process. Only a faint shell of residual bone is seen, indicating the superior vertebral body margins (small arrows). A large paraspinal inflammatory mass surrounds the infection (large arrows). The thoracic aorta (AO) is in close proximity to the discitis and spinal osteomyelitis.

Chapter 2 Neuroradiology Pearls _____

1. Caution: CT of the head done with contrast agents can obscure hemorrhage.
2. Patients with a leaking aneurysm as a cause of their SAH frequently complain of the "worst headache" they have ever experienced.
3. An isodense SDH can be difficult to diagnose on CT. Examine the scan for signs of mass effect. If the findings are equivocal, consider MRI.
4. "Clear" the cervical spine with cross-table radiographs prior to moving the patient or removing spine precautions.
5. Most cervical spine injuries in the pediatric population involve the C1 or C2 vertebrae. Pay careful attention to the synchondrosis at the base of the dens.
6. Cervical spine flexion-extension views are rarely of benefit in the acute setting and must be performed only by a cooperative, nonintoxicated patient without any assistance and only after the lateral cervical spine film has been cleared. Stop the exam immediately if the patient experiences pain or neurologic symptoms.
7. Pay close attention to the spinolaminal line on the lateral cervical spine film to avoid missing a C2 traumatic spondylolisthesis (hangman's fracture).
8. Multiple spine fractures are common.
9. Cervical spine fractures through the foramen transversarium (C3–C6) can injure the vertebral artery.
10. Carefully inspect the paraspinous tissue, adjacent to the thoracic spine, for any abnormal widening.
11. Always consider the possibility of lumbar vertebral body compression fractures when a patient falls and has suffered calcaneal fracture(s).
12. Examine lumbar spine radiographs for calcification and dilatation of the abdominal aorta. Patients with aortic dissections can present with back pain, which may be misinterpreted as musculoskeletal in origin.

Chapter

3

Chest

OVERVIEW

Patients who come to the emergency department with reports of either cardiac or pulmonary symptoms usually have screening posteroanterior (PA) and lateral chest radiographs taken as the initial step in their radiographic evaluation (Algorithm 3-1). Evaluating abnormal findings on chest radiographs can be extremely difficult, especially if the patient has a complex medical history. Consequently, it is important to obtain a thorough medical history and retrieve any previous chest radiographs for comparison. Evaluation of chest radiographs including a limited differential diagnosis of abnormal findings is included in Table 3-1.

TECHNIQUES

PA and Lateral Chest Radiography

This is the routine standard two-view screening examination for patients who can adequately cooperate and are not critically ill. It is important that the films be obtained with the patient in an upright position. Each film should be evaluated for technical quality in terms of positioning and technique. Rotational artifacts or poor technique can lead to difficulties in diagnosis. The differences between inspiration and expiration films are demonstrated in Figure 3-1.

ALGORITHM 3-1   Evaluation of the Patient with Cardiac or Pulmonary Symptoms

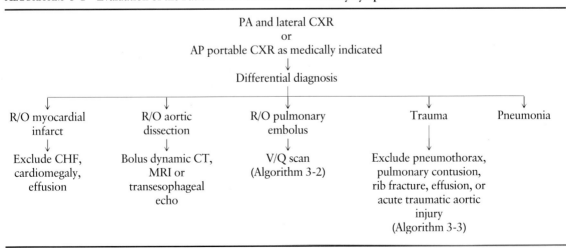

PA and lateral CXR
or
AP portable CXR as medically indicated
↓
Differential diagnosis

R/O myocardial infarct	R/O aortic dissection	R/O pulmonary embolus	Trauma	Pneumonia
↓	↓	↓	↓	
Exclude CHF, cardiomegaly, effusion	Bolus dynamic CT, MRI or transesophageal echo	V/Q scan (Algorithm 3-2)	Exclude pneumothorax, pulmonary contusion, rib fracture, effusion, or acute traumatic aortic injury (Algorithm 3-3)	

TABLE 3-1   Evaluation of Chest Radiographs

Structure	Radiographic Finding	Common Differential Diagnosis
Mediastinum	Shift	Atelectasis
		Postoperative volume loss
	Widening, > 8 cm	Vascular ectasia
		Neoplasm
		Post traumatic hematoma
		Inflammation; perforated esophagus, abscess
		Enlarged lymph nodes
Pulmonary hilum	Enlargement	Pulmonary artery enlargement, question COPD
		Pulmonary venous engorgement, CHF
		Enlarged lymph nodes, inflammatory/neoplastic
Heart	Enlarged cardiac silhouette	Cardiomegaly
		Pericardial effusion or tamponade
Pulmonary parenchyma	Opacities with volume loss	Atelectasis, obstruction large airways from neoplasm, mucous plug or endobronchial foreign body
	Lobar/segmental opacities	Pneumonia, #1 (see Table 3-5)
		Neoplasm
		Hemorrhage, exclude pulmonary emboli
	Confluent opacities	Pulmonary edema #1
		Pneumonia
		Hemorrhage
	Interstitial opacities	(See Table 3-4)
	Masses	Primary or metastatic neoplasm
		Infectious; fungal, i.e., histoplasmosis
	Focal hyperlucency	Absence of normal structures, i.e., mastectomy
		Blebs, question COPD
		Pneumothorax
	Global hyperluceny	Pneumothorax
Pleural space	Blunted costophrenic angles	Effusion (Table 3-7) vs. pleural thickening
Chest Wall	Fractures or bony abnormalities	
Diaphragm	Elevation	Subpulmonic effusion, #1
		Atelectasis
		Traumatic rupture

Portable AP Films

Critically ill patients or patients who cannot cooperate with the standard two-view chest examination commonly undergo portable radiography. This is usually limited to a single anteroposterior (AP) view. Portable AP films are technically limited because of magnification artifact, supine positioning, and poor patient cooperation (Figure 3-2). If possible, obtain erect AP films, as supine films are further degraded by poor inspiration and increased pulmonary blood volume.

Apical Lordotic View

This view is obtained by angling the tube cephalad to evaluate the lung apices. Not uncommonly, costochondral calcifications and bony structures obscure the apex of the lungs. Apical lordotic films project bony structures off the underlying parenchyma to allow better visualization (Figure 3-3).

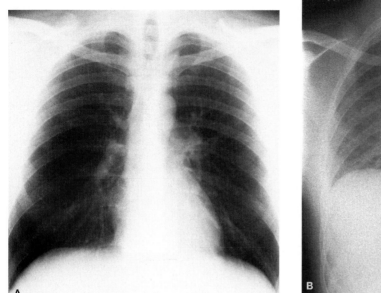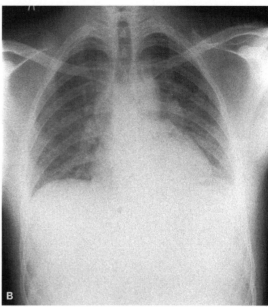

FIGURE 3-1 **Normal PA chest: Inspiration vs. expiration:** PA views of the same patient obtained the same day demonstrate the difference between radiographs obtained during deep inspiration (A) and expiration (B). Note in (B) that the heart appears large and the pulmonary vessels are engorged, simulating congestive heart failure.

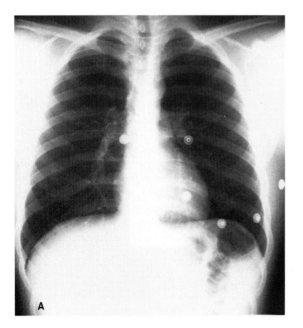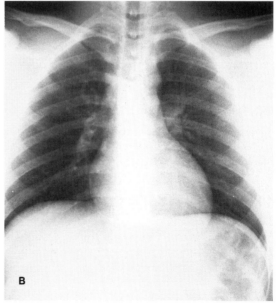

FIGURE 3-2 **Normal PA chest: Supine vs. erect position:** PA views of the same patient from the same day demonstrate the difference between radiographs obtained with the patient erect (A) and supine (B). In (B), the increase in pulmonary blood volume and effects of gravity simulate pulmonary venous hypertension and an enlarged heart.

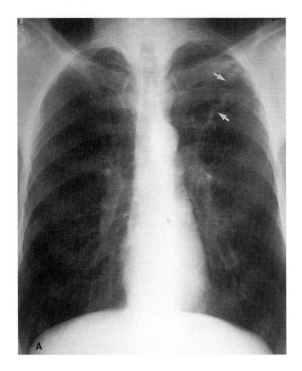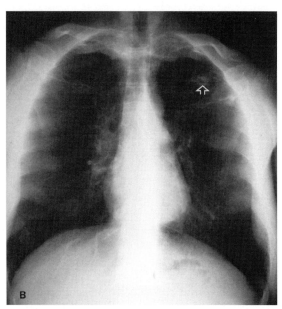

FIGURE 3-3   **PA and apical lordotic chest: Reactivation tuberculosis:** In (A), there is an ill-defined air-space process involving the left upper lobe (arrows). The apical lordotic view (B) demonstrates a small thick-walled cavity (open arrow) in this patient with reactivation tuberculosis.

Lateral Decubitus View

A lateral decubitus view of the chest is obtained to assess whether there is any free flowing pleural fluid in the dependent hemithorax. It is done by positioning patients on their side. For example, a left-lateral decubitus film is taken with the patient positioned on their left side. Lateral decubitus views are also obtained in evaluating the possibility of pediatric endobronchial foreign bodies.

Rib Series

When clinically necessary, additional oblique views of the chest utilizing bone technique may be advantageous in detecting rib fractures.

CHEST RADIOGRAPH EVALUATION: ADULT

Interpretation of chest radiographs requires a consistent and thorough approach. All of the following elements should be examined:

1. Symmetry of the diaphragms with inspection of the costophrenic angles, both laterally and posteriorly. While the hemidiaphragms may appear level, it is not unusual for the right hemidiaphragm to be slightly higher than the left.

2. The heart should be normally located and all borders should be clearly defined. Mediastinal structures likewise should be easily seen and have distinct borders.

3. The trachea should be midline and the right paratracheal stripe should measure less than 5 mm in width.

4. The superior mediastinal borders are formed by vascular structures and are slightly curved or straight on the right. The aortic knob on the left is normally well defined and less than 3 cm in size in a transverse diameter.

5. The normal pulmonary hilar structures should be easily identified. The left hilum is usually slightly higher than the right hilum. Hilar size is extremely variable. Abnormal hilar enlargement is best evaluated by comparison with the contralateral side or prior studies. Caution is advised when utilizing this approach as patients with lymphoma, sarcoidosis, or pulmonary artery hypertension can present with bilateral hilar enlargement.

6. Normal lung parenchyma should be lucent and only bronchovascular structures should be visible. Vascular structures should taper and become almost indistinct at the lung periphery.

7. The minor fissure is on the right side in most patients and is horizontal.

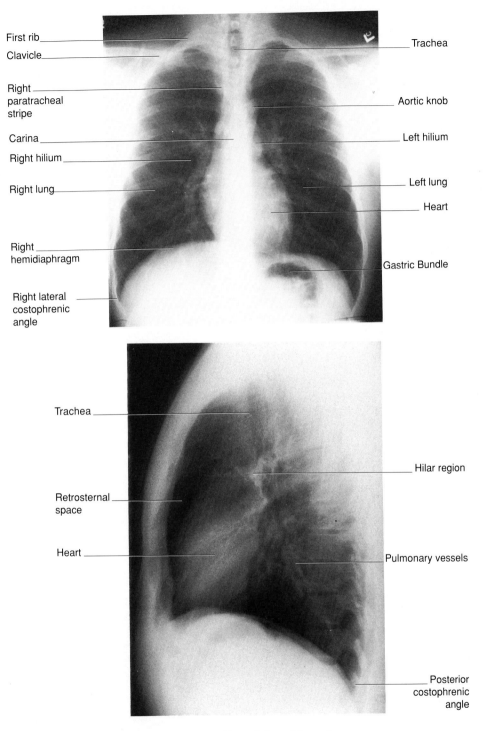

First rib

Clavicle

Right paratracheal stripe

Carina

Right hilium

Right lung

Right hemidiaphragm

Right lateral costophrenic angle

Trachea

Aortic knob

Left hilium

Left lung

Heart

Gastric Bundle

Trachea

Retrosternal space

Heart

Hilar region

Pulmonary vessels

Posterior costophrenic angle

FIGURE 3-4 **PA and lateral chest:** Normal anatomy

8. Major fissures are seen only on the lateral view and run in an oblique course from approximately the fifth thoracic vertebral body to the diaphragm.

9. The bony thorax should be inspected for rib fractures or bone lesions. A normal PA and lateral chest examination outlining normal anatomy is included in Figure 3-4.

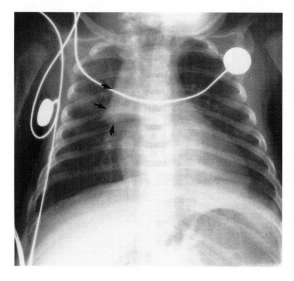

FIGURE 3-5 **AP newborn chest: Normal thymus:** Arrows indicate the border of the normal newborn thymus. This finding should not be confused with a pathologic process. Note the newborn heart occupies greater than half of the cardiothoracic ratio.

CHEST RADIOGRAPH EVALUATION: PEDIATRIC

Newborns have large thymus glands that normally widen the superior mediastinum. The right border of the thymus gland is angulated and resembles a boat's sail (Figure 3-5). The newborn heart is more globular in shape and occupies more than half of the cardiothoracic diameter. Newborn lungs are normally more lucent due to an underdeveloped interstitium.

Airway Obstruction

The differential diagnosis for acute infectious pediatric airway obstruction includes epiglottitis, croup, and retropharyngeal abscess. Emergency physicians frequently obtain radiographs to distinguish epiglottitis from croup (Figures 3-6, 3-7).

Epiglottitis and croup have very distinct differences in age group and etiologic organisms, although

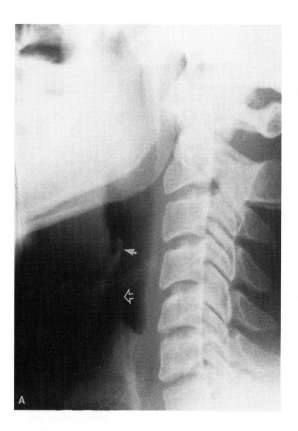

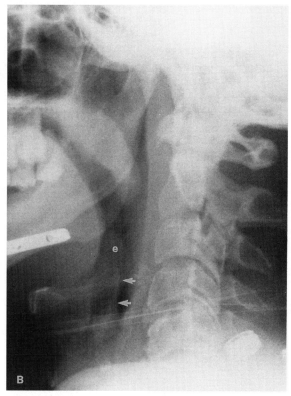

FIGURE 3-6 **Lateral soft tissue neck: Normal and epiglottitis:** (A) Normal anatomy: Epiglottis (arrow) and aryepiglottic folds (open arrow). (B) Adult epiglottitis: Thickening and swelling of the epiglottis (e) and aryepiglottic folds (arrows) indicate acute inflammation.

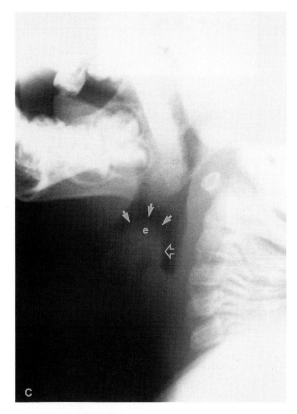

FIGURE 3-6 *(continued)*. (C) Pediatric epiglottitis: A large, swollen epiglottis (e) is present. Note that the inflamed epiglottis resembles an upward pointing thumb (arrows). Edematous aryepiglottic folds are visible (open arrow).

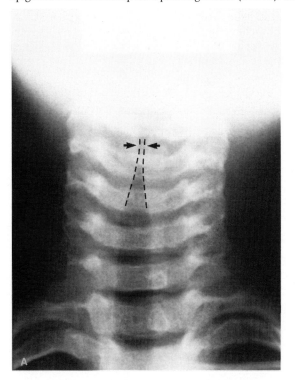

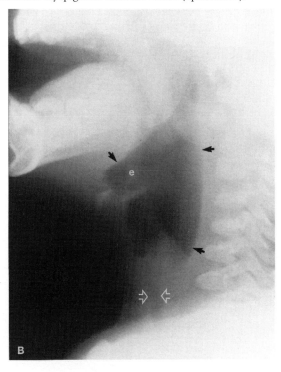

FIGURE 3-7 AP and lateral soft tissue neck: Croup: (A) AP view demonstrates narrowing of the glottic and subglottic airway (dashed lines and arrows). (B) Lateral view illustrates ballooning of the hypopharynx (arrows) and narrowing of the subglottic airway (open arrows). The epiglottis (e) and aryepiglottic folds are normal.

TABLE 3-2   Differential Diagnosis of Infectious Pediatric Airway Disease

	Epiglottitis[a]	Croup[b]	Retropharyngeal Abscess[c]
Patient Age	3–6 yrs	6 mos–3 yrs	Infants; young child
Organism	H. Influenza	Viral, parainfluenza/influenza	Many
Symptoms	Fever, inspiratory stridor, dysphagia	Barky cough inspiratory stridor	Fever, neck pain, dysphagia, enlarged cervical lymph nodes
Imaging Characteristics Soft Tissue View Lateral Neck	Enlarged epiglottis and aryepiglottic folds	Subglottic narrowing	Thickened retropharyngeal tissues. + presence of gas
Other	Medical emergency **Do Not** leave child unattended	History of antecedent lower respiratory tract infection	History of URI
	Drooling child		Barium swallow, anterior displacement of esophagus

[a]See Figure 3-6.
[b]See Figure 3-7.
[c]See Figure 3-8.

some overlap does exist (Table 3-2). Epiglottitis is a true medical emergency, and when the clinical diagnosis is suspected, a physician experienced in control of the pediatric airway should be in attendance with the patient at all times. While epiglottitis is most commonly seen in the pediatric population, adults too can present with acute epiglottitis. A retropharyngeal abscess can mimic epiglottitis and is included in the differential diagnosis of infectious pediatric airway diseases (Figure 3-8).

Categories of Parenchymal Disease

Parenchymal disease can be divided into four broad categories; alveolar air-space disease, interstitial disease, atelectasis, and parenchymal masses.

Alveolar disease is commonly manifested by parenchymal opacities with ill-defined borders that tend to coalesce and form air bronchograms. An air bronchogram is detected when air within intrapulmonary bronchi is seen surrounded by an abnormal parenchymal opacity (Figure 3-9).

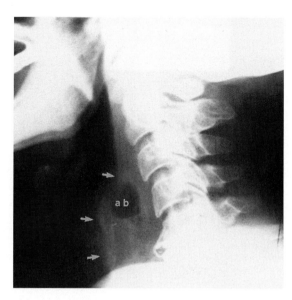

FIGURE 3-8   Lateral soft tissue neck: Retropharyngeal abscess: The airway is displaced anteriorly (arrows) by a large retropharyngeal abscess (ab). The retropharyngeal tissues are thickened and gas is present in the abscess.

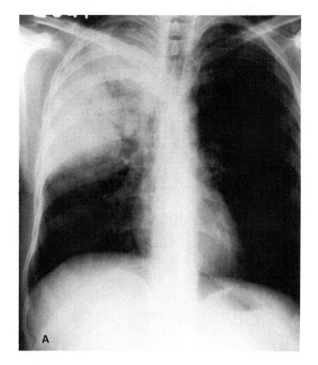

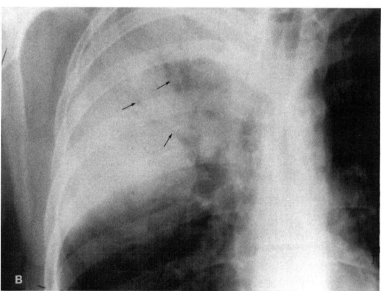

FIGURE 3-9 **PA chest and detail view right upper lobe: Klebsiella pneumonia:** (A) Marked consolidation of the right upper lobe is present in this patient with Klebsiella pneumonia. (B) Detail view demonstrates the characteristic air bronchograms (arrows) seen as the alveoli fill with inflammatory debris but the bronchi remain air filled.

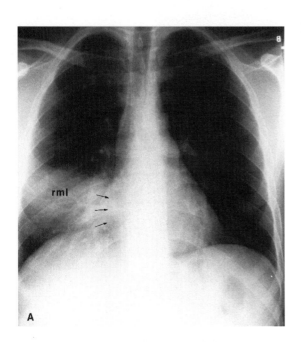
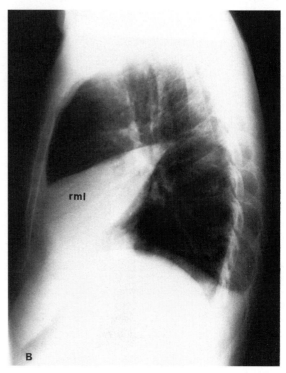

FIGURE 3-10 **PA and lateral chest: Right middle lobe pneumonia:** (A) PA view demonstrates air-space disease obscuring the right heart border silhouette (arrows). This silhouette sign indicates a medial segment pneumonia of the right middle lobe (rml). (B) Lateral view reveals the characteristic wedge-shaped consolidation seen with a right middle lobe pneumonia. This confirms the findings seen on the PA view.

Normal intrathoracic structures may be obscured by the presence of consolidative air-space disease. This is known as a silhouette sign. When the silhouette of the heart borders or the diaphragm is obscured by parenchymal opacities, this helps locate the segment(s) of diseased lung. If the right heart border is obscured, then the disease is located in the middle lobe (Figure 3-10). If either hemidiaphragm is obscured, then the disease is located in the lower lobe.

Differential diagnosis for alveolar air-space disease includes alveolar filling from water, blood, pus, or cells (Table 3-3).

Interstitial disease is an increase in opacity of the interstitial structures due to either acute or chronic causes. (Table 3-4) The predominant pattern may be linear, reticular, nodular, or a combination of the three. Like alveolar disease, interstitial processes can be either focal or diffuse. A brief differential diagnosis of interstitial diseases includes infection (Figure 3-11), fibrosis, pulmonary edema (Figure 3-30), and lymphangetic carcinomatosis (Figure 3-12).

Not uncommonly, interstitial processes have alveolar components and vice versa. Therefore, a mixed appearance on chest radiographs is common.

TABLE 3-3 **Differential Diagnosis of Alveolar Air Space Disease**

Acute	Chronic
Blood: Pulmonary hemorrhage, pulmonary contusion, vasculitis	"Goo": Alveolar proteinosis
Pus: Pneumonia	Cells: Bronchoalveolar carcinoma Lymphoma
Water: Pulmonary edema[a]	

[a]See Table 3-6.

TABLE 3-4   Differential Diagnosis of Interstitial Air Space Disease

Acute	Chronic

Pneumonia
  Viral
  Mycoplasma
  P. Carinii
 	
Hypersensitivity pneumonitis
 	
Congestive heart failure
	Lymphangitic carcinomatosis
	  Bronchogenic cancer
	  Metastatic breast cancer
	
	Collagen vascular disease
	  Scleroderma
	  Rheumatoid lung
	
	Miliary infection
	  Tuberculosis
	  Fungal disease
	
	Granulomatous disease
	  Sarcoid
	
	Drug reaction
	  Amiodarone
	  Methotrexate
	  Nitrofurantoin
	
	Idiopathic pulmonary fibrosis
	
	Pneumoconiosis
	  Silica
	  Coal workers' lung

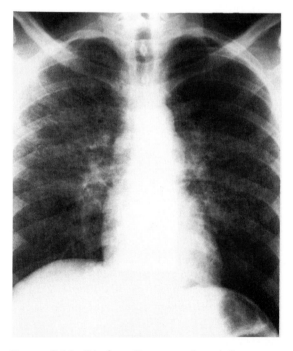

FIGURE 3-11   PA chest: *Pneumocystis carinii* pneumonia: This AIDS patient has a diffuse interstitial process that is worse in the upper lobes. Further testing diagnosed *P. carinii* pneumonia. A viral or atypical bacterial pneumonia would be suspected in a nonimmunocompromised patient.

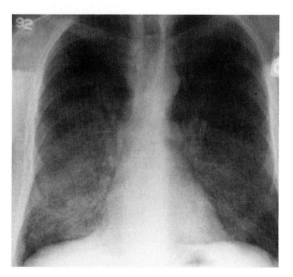

FIGURE 3-12   PA chest: Lymphangitic carcinomatosis: Bilateral predominately lower-lobe interstitial disease is present in this patient who presented to the emergency department complaining of shortness of breath. He died 2 weeks later, and lymphangitic spread of melanoma was found at autopsy. Two years earlier, the patient had a malignant mole excised from his back.

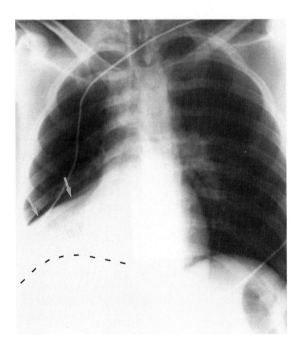

FIGURE 3-13   **PA chest: Right middle- and lower-lobe atelectasis:** The minor fissure is displaced inferiorly (arrows) secondary to volume loss of the right-middle and lower lobes. The collapsed lobes are opaque and obscure both the right heart border and right hemidiaphragm (silhouette sign). Ipsilateral shift of the mediastinum is an indirect sign that atelectasis is present.

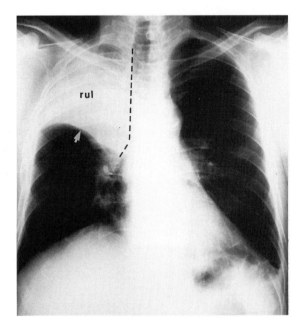

FIGURE 3-14   **PA chest: Right upper lobe atelectasis:** Collapse of the right upper lobe (rul) has obscured the right tracheal border (dashed lines) and elevated the minor fissure (arrow).

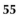

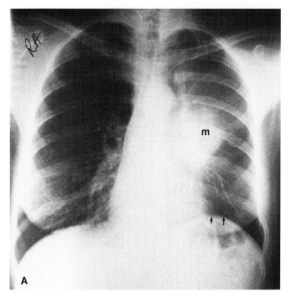

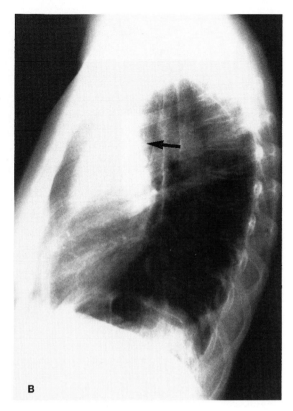

FIGURE 3-15 **PA and lateral chest: Left upper lobe atelectasis secondary to bronchogenic carcinoma:** (A) PA view demonstrates a left hilar mass (m). The mass is causing volume loss made evident by elevation of the left hemidiaphragm (arrows) and a subtle increase in opacity of the left hemithorax. (B) Lateral projection reveals the atelectatic left upper lobe as an anterior opacity (arrow).

Atelectasis, also known as regional or localized lung collapse or volume loss, is classified according to the etiology. Radiographically, the best indicator for volume loss is displacement of the interlobar fissures (Figures 3-13, 3-14). Collapsed lung segments appear opaque and may also present as a silhouette sign. Volume loss is also associated with a shift of the mediastinum toward the collapse. Other indirect signs of atelectasis include hilar displacement toward the collapsed segment(s) and ipsilateral elevation of the hemidiaphragm.

The two categories of atelectasis the emergency physician encounters most are obstructive and passive. Obstructive atelectasis is secondary to endobronchial obstruction. Common forms of obstruction are mucus plugs, foreign bodies, bronchogenic carcinoma (Figure 3-15), or iatrogenic causes such as misplaced endotracheal tubes (Figure 3-16). Passive atelectasis is due to mass effect on the lung from either fluid from a large pleural effusion or air from a pneumothorax.

Parenchymal masses can be single (Figures 3-17, 3-18) or multiple (Figure 3-19) and are commonly due to primary or metastatic neoplastic disease. Septic emboli, vasculitis, and fungal disease can also cause pulmonary nodules. Occasionally, if an isolated spherical opacity is identified, round pneumonia may be the cause (Figure 3-20).

A benign mass is one that demonstrates characteristic central dense calcification of granulomatous disease (Figure 3-21) or has demonstrated no growth over a two-year period.

Most pulmonary masses require further evaluation with CT and, possibly, needle biopsy to obtain a diagnosis. Of primary concern is bronchogenic carcinoma. Radiographs should be evaluated for associated adenopathy, pleural effusion, and bone destruction.

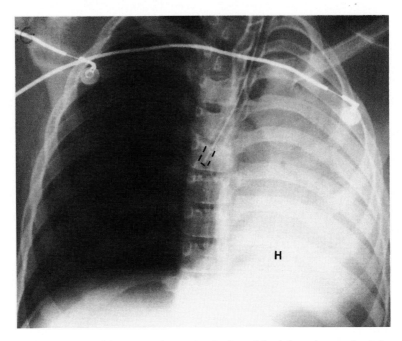

FIGURE 3-16   **AP chest: Collapsed left lung secondary to intubation of the right main-stem bronchus:** The endotracheal tube tip (dashed lines) is in the right main-stem bronchus. The left lung has collapsed resulting in complete opacification of the left hemithorax. The heart (H) borders are completely obscured. The volume loss has shifted the trachea and mediastinal structures to the left. Such shifting is an important diagnostic key to distinguish atelectasis from a large pleural effusion which would cause contralateral mediastinal shift.

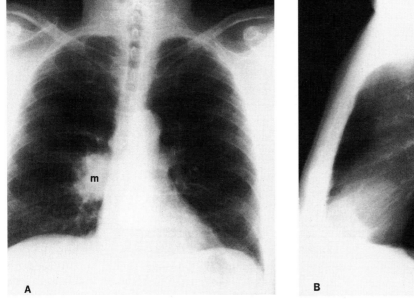
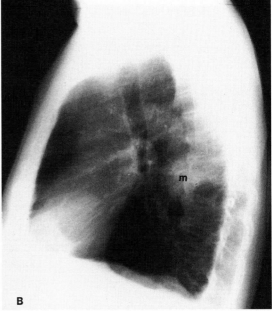

FIGURE 3-17   **PA and lateral chest: Bronchogenic carcinoma:** A large ill-defined mass (m) is projecting into the right infrahilar area on the PA view (A). The lateral projection (B) demonstrates the mass (m) to be posterior in location.

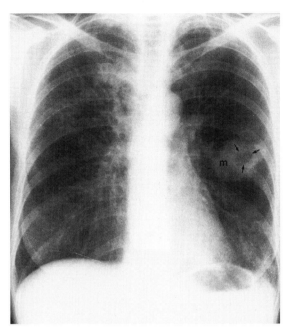

FIGURE 3-18 PA chest: Cavitary squamous cell carcinoma: A mass (m) with a central cavity (arrows) is visible in the left mid-chest. The cavity formed secondary to tissue necrosis. Necrosis and cavitation most commonly occur either from neoplastic disease or a lung abscess.

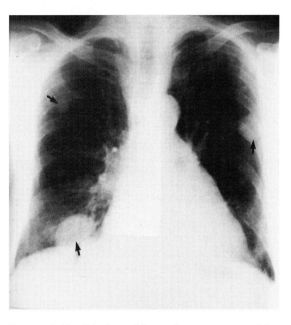

FIGURE 3-19 PA chest: Metastatic osteosarcoma: Numerous well-defined metastatic lesions of varying sizes are scattered throughout the chest (arrows). Metastatic colon and renal cell carcinoma can have a similar appearance.

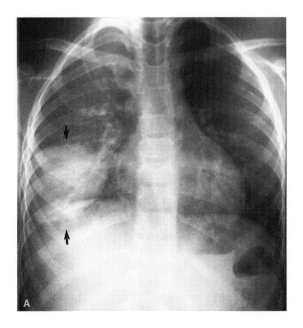

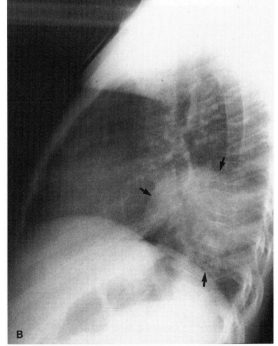

FIGURE 3-20 PA and lateral chest: Round pneumonia: This child presented with a fever and cough. (A) The PA view reveals a large right lower lobe mass (arrows). (B) On lateral projection, the mass is well-defined (arrows). Round pneumonias are typically caused by pneumococcus and represent an early consolidative process. The key to the diagnosis is the clinical presentation and radiographic follow-up.

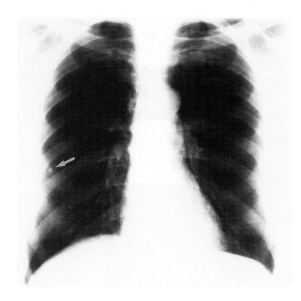

←

FIGURE 3-21 **PA chest: Calcified granuloma:** A small densely calcified granuloma is in the right lateral mid-chest (arrow). Calcification within a pulmonary nodule is a reliable indicator that the nodule is benign. Common granulomatous infections causing parenchymal (as well as nodal) calcifications include histoplasmosis, tuberculosis, and coccidioidomycosis. In addition to granulomas, hamartomas frequently calcify.

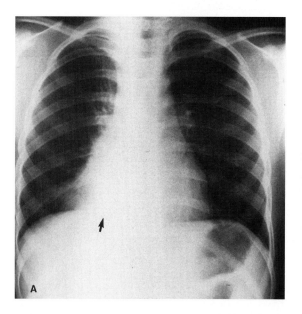

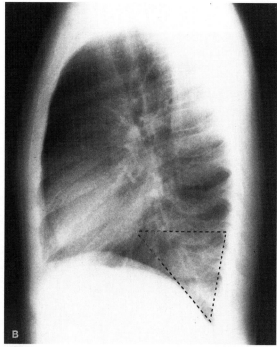

FIGURE 3-22 **PA and lateral chest: Right lower lobe pneumonia:** (A) PA view demonstrates consolidation obscuring the right medial hemidiaphragm (arrow). (B) Lateral view reveals retrocardiac opacification (dashed triangle). It is an important diagnostic key to remember that the spine becomes more lucent as one proceeds from cephalad to caudal on the lateral projection. Any opacity in this area, however subtle, requires careful consideration.

TABLE 3-5   Community Acquired Pneumonia Etiologic Agents: Patients at Risk

Radiographic findings	Noncompromised	Immunocompromised, Non-HIV	Immunocompromised: HIV positive; AIDS
Lobar consolidation— Alveolar air space disease (Figure 3-9)	*Streptococcus pneumoniae* *Klebsiella*; Alcoholics *Staph. aureus*; IVDA bacterial endocarditis, secondary pneumonia after viral infection *Legionella pneumophila* *Hemophilus influenzae*; COPD, alcoholics	Gram negative organism *Klebsiella* *Pseudomonas* *E. coli* *Legionella*; Renal transplant patients *Staph. aureus*	*M. tuberculosis* Bacteria *Staph. aureus* *H. influenza* *P. carinii*
Nodular densities (Figure 3-24)	Varicella pneumonia; small, scattered nodules	Bacterial; *Nocardia* Fungal; *Aspergillus, Cryptococcus*	*M. tuberculosis* Fungi; *Cryptococcus,* Histoplasmosis
Consolidation with cavitation (necrotizing pneumonia) (Figure 3-25)	Gram negative organisms secondary to aspiration *Klebsiella* *E. coli* Anaerobes *S. pneumoniae* *Staph. aureus*	Gram negative organisms *Aspergillus*	*Nocardia* Gram negative organism
Upper lobe consolidation + cavitation (Figure 3-3, 3-28)	*M. tuberculosis*	*M. tuberculosis*	*P. carinii* treated with pentamidine *M. tuberculosis* *M. kansasii*
Ill-defined air space opacities (bronchopneumonia) (Figure 3-26)	*Staph. aureus* Gram negative Bacteria *M. Tuberculosis*		
Interstitial disease (Figure 3-11)	*Mycoplasma pneumoniae* Viral	*P. carinii* Viral: Herpes CMV: Organ transplant recipients	*P. carinii* CMV
Consolidation with pleural effusion and lymphadenopathy	Anaerobes *M. tuberculosis* (Also think lung CA)	*M. tuberculosis*	*M. tuberculosis*

Note: CXR may be normal in AIDS patients with *P. carinii* and disseminated fungal disease.

Pneumonia

Chest radiographs are frequently ordered by the emergency physician to exclude the possibility of pneumonia. Typical radiographic features of pneumonia are areas of pulmonary consolidation (Figure 3-9). These may be isolated or multiple depending on the infective agent. Some may show cavitation, and there may be an associated parapneumonic effusion.

The radiographic presentation of pneumonia is highly variable (Figures 3-22, 3-23). Infective agents, age of patient, status of the patient's immune system, and preexisting disease all influence the appearance of chest radiographs.

Radiographically, it is not possible to determine the exact etiologic agent causing the symptoms of pneumonia. It is useful, however, to categorize the radiographic findings according to their appearance, the patient's immune status, and risk factors (Table 3-5). Almost all pneumonias encountered in the emergency department are community, rather than hospital, acquired.

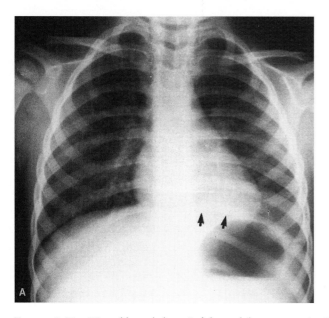

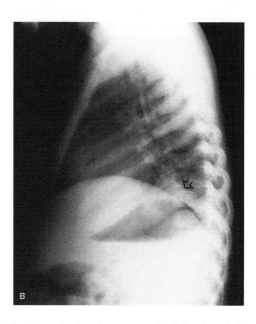

FIGURE 3-23   PA and lateral chest: Left lower lobe pneumonia: (A) The PA projection shows a poorly defined medial left hemidiaphragm (arrows). (B) The lateral film demonstrates retrocardiac opacification (open arrow) indicating this early pneumonia.

Multiple gram-positive and gram-negative bacteria, as well as numerous viruses and fungi, are etiologic agents of pneumonia. Adenoviruses as well as herpes viruses are the two major groups of DNA viruses that cause lower respiratory tract infections. Early in the course of a viral pneumonia, an interstitial process predominates. The inflammatory process may ultimately produce patchy air-space consolidation, usually representing atelectasis. Other viruses that have pulmonary sequela include the varicella virus, measles virus, influenza virus, and in the pediatric population, respiratory syncytial virus.

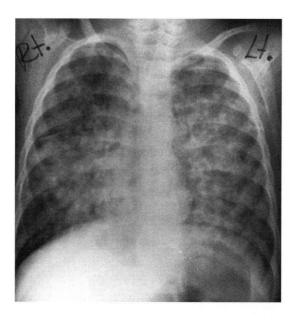

FIGURE 3-24   AP chest: Varicella pneumonia: Numerous bilateral, ill-defined nodular opacities are seen in this child with varicella pneumonia. Patients who are immunocompromised are at greatest risk for developing pulmonary complications from this common disease.

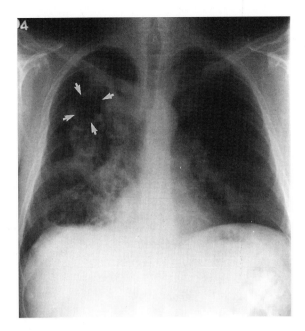

FIGURE 3-25   AP chest: Nocardia pneumonia: A homogenous, nonsegmental consolidative air-space process is present in the right chest. Numerous cavities are distributed throughout the parenchymal opacities, the largest in the upper lobe (arrows). This is a case of necrotizing pneumonia caused by nocardia.

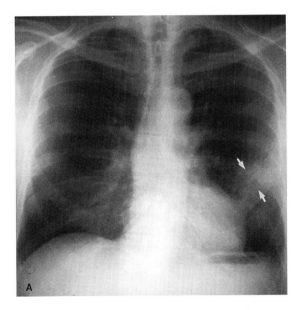
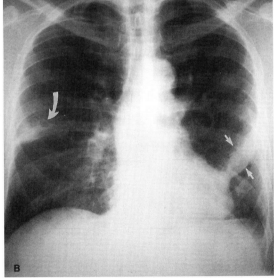

FIGURE 3-26   PA chest: Bronchopneumonia: This 40-year-old male presented to the emergency department (ED) with lower respiratory complaints. (A) The initial radiograph revealed an ill-defined air-space process in the left upper lobe (arrows). The patient was started on antibiotics but returned to the ED two days later with worsening symptoms. (B) The follow-up chest radiograph demonstrates the left upper lobe consolidation (arrows) as well as a new focus of air-space disease in the right upper lobe (curved arrow). These findings are characteristic of a bronchopneumonia.

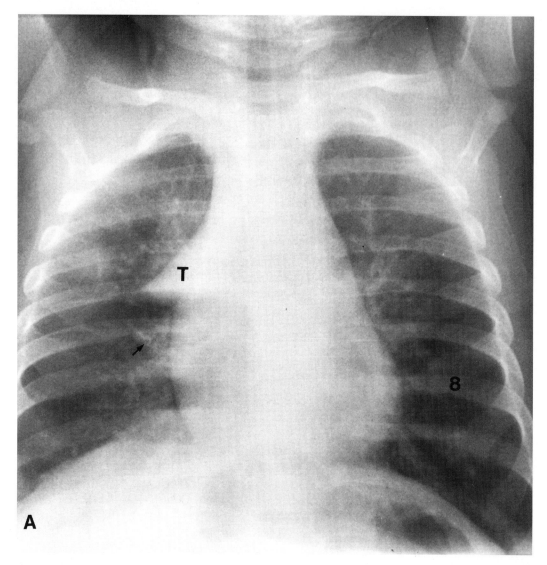

FIGURE 3-27 **PA and lateral chest: Viral bronchiolitis :** Young child with respiratory symptoms. (A) The PA view demonstrates greater than eight posterior ribs of inflation (8). This finding indicates air trapping and hyperinflation. The bronchi are thick walled (arrow). The normal thymus (T) is visible.

Lower respiratory tract infection in the pediatric population is usually due to viral causes. Chest radiographs demonstrate bilateral air trapping with hyperinflation and peribronchial thickening (Figure 3-27). Air-space disease seen in association with hyperinflation and peribronchial cuffing usually represents superimposed atelectasis. The differential diagnosis for the above findings is between viral bronchiolitis and reactive airways disease.

In AIDS patients, *Pneumocystis carinii* is the most common pathogen encountered in patients with pulmonary symptoms. *P. carinii* can present as an interstitial (Figure 3-11) or fulminative alveolar consolidative process. Symptomatic patients, however, may present with normal chest radiographs. An association exists between HIV-infected patients and pulmonary tuberculosis. Tuberculosis should be suspected in HIV-positive patients when diffuse interstitial lung disease is seen in conjunction with hilar or mediastinal adenopathy.

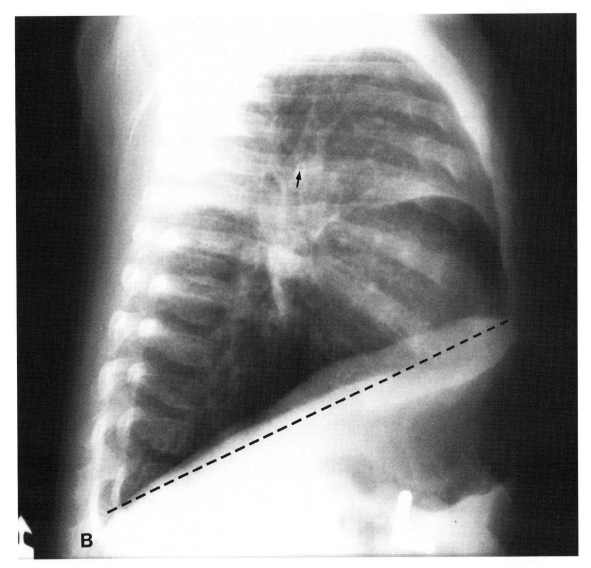

FIGURE 3-27 Continued. (B) On the lateral view the diaphragms are flattened, an additional sign of air trapping. More thick-walled bronchi are visible (arrow). Although this is a case of viral bronchiolitis, a child with asthma could have similar findings.

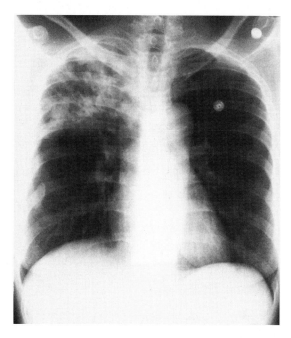

FIGURE 3-28   **PA chest: Reactivation tuberculosis:** An inhomogeneous air-space process involving the right upper lobe is visible. Reactivation or postprimary tuberculosis commonly involves the apical and posterior segments of the right upper lobe. More than half of these cases demonstrate cavitation. Lymph node enlargement is uncommon.

Tuberculosis

The incidence of pulmonary tuberculosis has been steadily increasing and is becoming a major public health issue in many large cities. Of primary concern is the emergence of drug-resistant tuberculosis. Primary tuberculosis usually presents radiographically with homogenous consolidation without cavitation. This can involve either upper or lower lobes and may also present with adenopathy. In a pediatric patient, adenopathy and air-space disease should equate to tuberculosis until proven otherwise. The majority of patients infected with primary pulmonary tuberculosis have no clinical evidence of disease and may present with mild nonspecific symptoms.

Reactivation tuberculosis characteristically involves the apices or posterior segments of the upper lobes (Figure 3-28). Cavitation in association with air-space disease is a common finding (Figure 3-3).

Pulmonary Edema

Alveolar filling from pulmonary edema is most commonly seen in the emergency department sec-ondary to left ventricular failure and increasing pulmonary venous pressures. The congestive heart failure patient proceeds through a spectrum of radiographic findings, depending on the severity of the disease and acuity of symptoms. Initially, the patient presents with redistribution of the pulmonary venous blood flow to the apices of the lungs. This is also known as pulmonary venous cephalization. As the pulmonary venous pressure continues to increase, interstitial congestion occurs next. Radiographically, this presents as prominence of the interstitium with ill-defined vascular walls, peribronchial cuffing, and Kerley-B lines. Kerley-B lines are parallel fine lines extending from the pleural surface into the subpleural lung. These lines represent thickening of the interlobular septa and are most commonly seen at the lung base (Figure 3-29). Continuing along the spectrum of disease, as the pulmonary venous pressures rise, fluid begins to fill the alveoli, creating a perihilar bat wing or butterfly pattern of air-space disease (Figure 3-30). This is usually bilaterally symmetrical but may present atypically due to underlying lung disease or positional variation and gravitational effects (Figure 3-31).

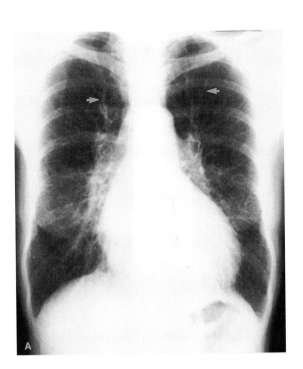
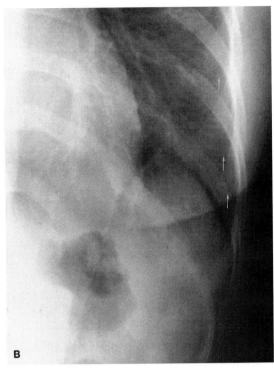

FIGURE 3-29 **PA chest and detail view of left lung base: Congestive heart failure with Kerley-B lines:** (A) PA view demonstrates an enlarged cardiac silhouette. There is pulmonary venous hypertension with cephalization (large arrows). (B) The detail view reveals fine parallel lines extending from the pleural surface (small arrows). These Kerley-B lines represent thickening of the interlobular septa. No evidence of alveolar air-space disease is seen and no effusions are identified. The above findings may represent a patient with chronic compensated heart failure or early acute CHF.

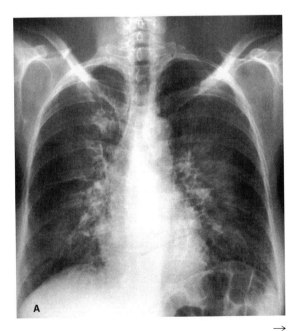
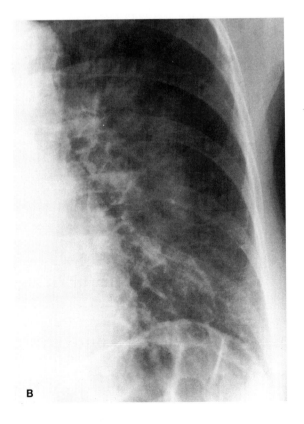

$\rightarrow$

FIGURE 3-30 **PA chest and detail view of the left base: Acute CHF:** (A) The PA view reveals inhomogeneous air-space disease centrally obscuring the hilar structures. This is more visible on the detailed view (B). Fluid is filling the alveoli and creating a perihilar bat wing appearance.

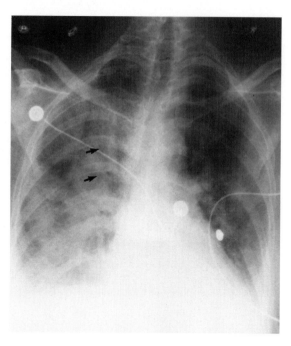

Figure 3-31 **AP chest: Dependent pulmonary edema:** Single view of the chest demonstrates bilateral areas of consolidation with sparing of the left upper lobe. There are numerous air bronchograms in the right chest representing alveolar fluid secondary to congestive heart failure (arrows). The asymmetry seen on the radiograph can be explained by gravitational effects as the patient preferentially lies on the right side.

Other causes of pulmonary edema are due to increased vascular permeability and include toxic inhalation, drug overdose, renal failure, and sepsis (Table 3-6). These present with radiographic findings similar to those seen with left ventricular failure (Figure 3-32).

Adult respiratory distress syndrome (ARDS) is a severe form of noncardiac pulmonary edema. Damaged pulmonary capillaries with impaired surfactant production result in fluid leaking into the pulmonary interstitium and alveoli. Radiographically, ARDS appears as a diffuse interstitial/alveolar airspace process that becomes more confluent with time (see Figure 3-68).

TABLE 3-6   **Noncardiac Causes of Pulmonary Edema**

Chronic renal failure: Uremia

Drug overdose: Heroin, salicylates

Toxic inhalation: Smoke, NO_2, SO_2, chlorine, ammonia

High altitude

Neurogenic causes

Sepsis

Near-drowning

Shock

Burn injuries

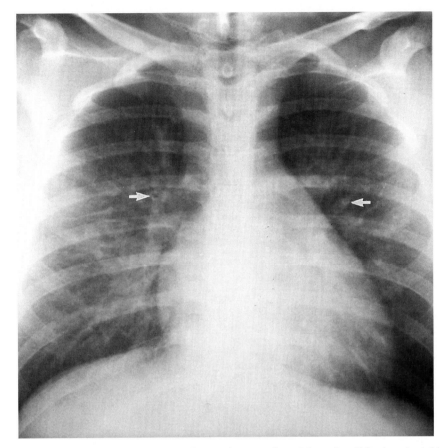

FIGURE 3-32   **AP chest: Pulmonary edema secondary to drug overdose:** Bilateral perihilar haze is visible in conjunction with peribronchial cuffing (arrows). Fluid has transudated into the peribronchovascular space resulting in poor definition of the pulmonary vascular markings. This patient had increased capillary permeability from a heroin overdose.

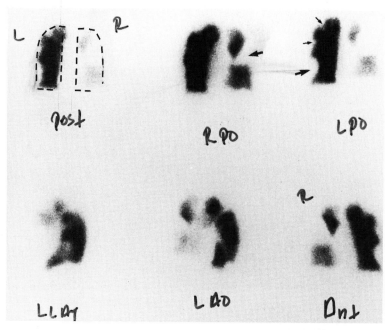

FIGURE 3-33 **Perfusion images from a V/Q scan: High probability for pulmonary emboli:** This perfusion scan is markedly abnormal. There are a number of peripheral wedge-shaped areas of absent perfusion (arrows). Many of these are segmental in size, whereas others are subsegmental. These findings, combined with a normal ventilation scan, represent a high probability (85%) for pulmonary emboli.

Pulmonary Embolism

Untreated pulmonary thromboembolic disease is associated with a high mortality. Unfortunately, because chest radiographs are commonly normal they are of little assistance. Findings, such as parenchymal consolidation, pleural effusion, and focal areas of oligemia, are nonspecific.

Nuclear medicine ventilation perfusion scans (V-Q scans) are the initial screening test to detect pulmonary emboli. Chest radiographs are an important component in accurately interpreting V-Q scans as well as excluding other pulmonary disease and should be obtained prior to consulting nuclear medicine. The hallmark of pulmonary emboli on a V-Q scan are areas that have normal ventilation but abnormal perfusion (Figure 3-33).

V-Q scans are interpreted as normal, low, intermediate, or high, regarding the probability of pulmonary emboli. A normal ventilation perfusion scan essentially excludes pulmonary emboli. A low-probability scan has a less than 10% chance of pulmonary embolic disease. If the scan is high in probability, there is an 85% chance that the patient has pulmonary embolic disease. Unfortunately, intermediate ventilation perfusion results only correlate to a 50–50 chance of pulmonary embolic disease.

Clinical suspicion is important when interpreting V/Q results and considering additional diagnostic tests (see Algorithm 3-2). The gold standard in the diagnosis of pulmonary emboli is the pulmonary angiogram that demonstrates thrombus in the pulmonary arteries (Figure 3-34).

Approximately 30% of patients with pulmonary emboli have concurrent deep vein thrombosis (DVT). The patient with DVT may have calf swelling and redness. Patients commonly report periods of prolonged sitting or bed rest prior to becoming symptomatic. Other risk factors include estrogen use, cancer, pregnancy, cardiac arrhythmia, and clotting disorders. The diagnosis can be made with contrast venography, which can demonstrate intraluminal clot in the deep venous system (Figure 3-35). Noninvasive diagnosis with Doppler ultrasound will demonstrate noncompressability of the deep thrombotic veins (Figure 3-36).

Patients with recent (24 to 72 hours) long-bone fractures, especially femur and tibia, are at risk for fat embolism. Fat particles disseminate throughout the body and the resulting emboli can cause neurologic and respiratory symptoms. Chest radiographs usually demonstrate nonspecific air-space opacities that tend to be peripheral and more common in the lower lobes.

ALGORITHM 3-2   Evaluation of the Patient with Suspected Pulmonary Emboli

Suspected pulmonary emboli
    ↓
Start IV heparin unless
contraindicated
    ↓

V/Q Scan	→	Low probability 10%	+	Low clinical suspicion	→	Stop heparin
			+	Moderate or high clinical suspicion	→	Continue heparin: rule-out deep vein thrombosis (R/O DVT)
	→	Intermediate probability 50%	+	Low clinical suspicion	→	Continue heparin: R/O DVT or entertain another diagnosis
			+	High clinical suspicion	→	Continue heparin, R/O DVT or pulmonary angiography
	→	High probability 85%	→			Continue heparin, consider IVC filter if heparin contraindicated

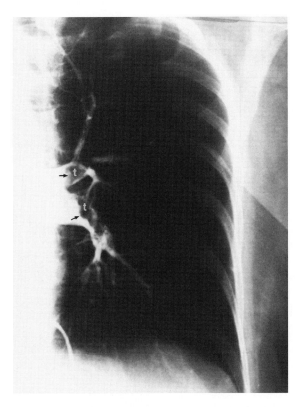

FIGURE 3-34   **Detail view left upper lobe pulmonary angiogram: Pulmonary emboli:** Thrombus (t) is visible in the left pulmonary arteries (arrows). These pulmonary emboli are outlined by contrast that was injected into the main pulmonary artery.

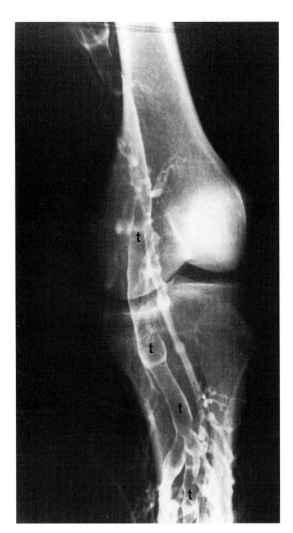

←

FIGURE 3-35 **Lower extremity venogram: Deep vein thrombosis (DVT):** Thrombus (t) is present throughout the deep veins of the calf and the popliteal fossa, and extends cephalad. The thin line of contrast outlining this extensive DVT is from an injection into a dorsal foot vein.

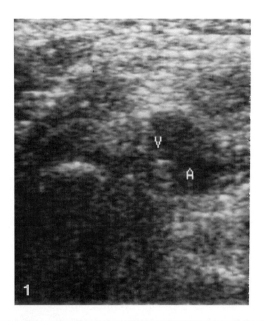

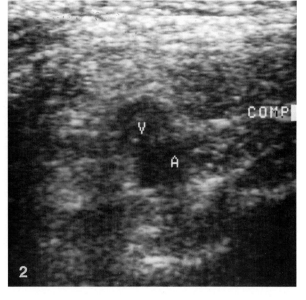

→

FIGURE 3-36 **Lower extremity venous ultrasound: DVT:** (1) Represents imaging of the deep femoral vein (v) without compression. The femoral artery (A) is seen adjacent to the vein. Imaging of the same area with compression (2) shows the vein to be unchanged in size. A normal vessel would easily compress with external transducer pressure and would no longer be visible. This noncompressibility results from a vein that is filled with thrombus.

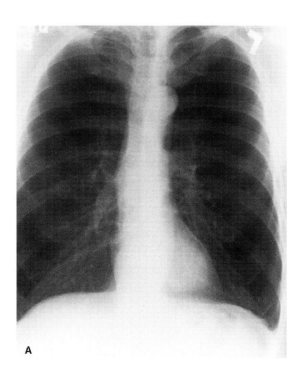

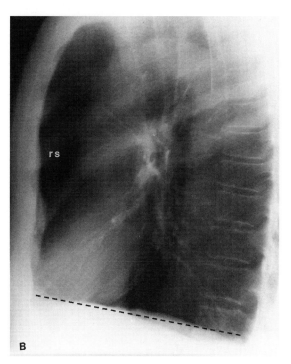

FIGURE 3-37 **PA and lateral chest: COPD:** Two standard views of the chest demonstrate the stigmata of obstructive lung disease. (A) On the PA the lungs appear lucent, suggesting air trapping and hyperinflation. (B) This is confirmed on the lateral by flattened hemidiaphragms (dashed line). The retrosternal space (rs) is increased as the hyperinflated lungs herniate anteriorly across the midline.

Chronic Obstructive Pulmonary Disease (COPD)

COPD refers to either chronic bronchitis or emphysema. The diagnosis of chronic obstructive pulmonary disease is not made from chest radiographs, but with pulmonary function tests. Chest radiographs, however, can have characteristic findings including flattening of the hemidiaphragms, increased lung volume with increased AP diameter of the thorax, and an increased retrosternal space indicative of the herniation of the hyperinflated lungs across the midline (Figure 3-37). Alterations in size and position of the normal pulmonary blood vessels suggest underlying bullous disease or blebs (Figure 3-38).

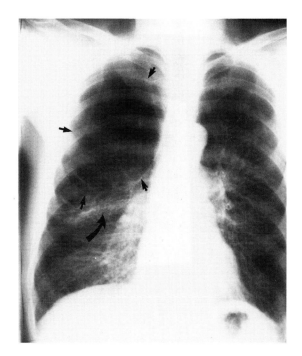

$\rightarrow$

FIGURE 3-38 **PA chest: COPD with large apical bleb:** A focal hyperlucency involving the right upper lung (arrows) is visible. This represents a large bleb. The normal bronchovascular structures are displaced inferiorly and appear as a linear opacity in the mid chest (curved arrow).

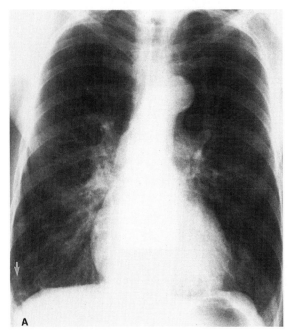

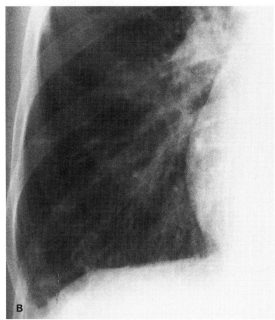

FIGURE 3-39   PA chest and detail view right base: COPD complicated by CHF: (A) PA view reveals hyperlucency of the chest in this patient with COPD. The cardiac silhouette is large, and there are Kerley-B lines at the right base (arrow). (B) Detail view illustrates the interstitial changes and poor vascular definition frequently seen with CHF. The findings are not bilaterally symmetric, a common occurrence in obstructive lung disease.

Chest radiographs are important for excluding complications when evaluating patients with known COPD who report to the emergency department with increasing shortness of breath. These complications include pneumonia, pulmonary edema, pulmonary artery hypertension, pneumothorax, as well as bronchogenic carcinoma. Caution is warranted as patients with COPD can present with atypical radiographic findings for pneumonia or pulmonary edema (Figure 3-39).

BRONCHIAL FOREIGN BODIES

Inhalation of radiopaque foreign bodies usually presents no diagnostic dilemma, as they are readily apparent on radiographs (Figure 3-40). However, nonradiopaque substances, such as peanuts, can cause difficulty in diagnosis. The radiographic diagnosis is made by demonstrating inappropriate air trapping. If the patient is cooperative, chest films obtained in full expiration demonstrate air trapping as increased lucency and hyperinflation of the affected hemithorax. Another sign of air trapping is shift of the mediastinum to the contralateral side. If the patient is too young to adequately cooperate with expiratory chest views, chest fluoroscopy or even lateral decubitus views may be of benefit. When lateral decubitus views are obtained, the dependent side is considered to be the expiratory view equivalent and will remain expanded and hyperlucent with endobronchial obstruction. It is important to obtain both left and right lateral decubitus views for comparison purposes.

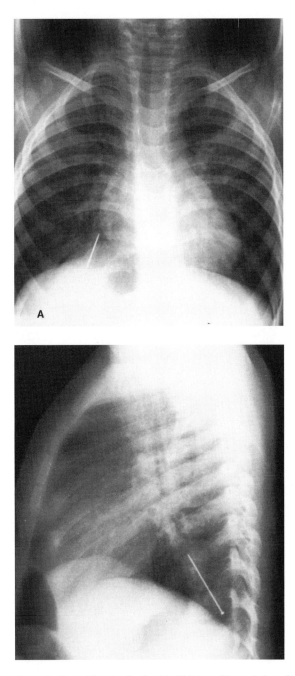

FIGURE 3-40 PA and lateral chest: Aspirated foreign body: (A, B) PA and lateral chest films of this young patient who aspirated a straight pin demonstrates the foreign body lodged in the posterior right lower lobe. Aspiration of radiopaque objects usually presents no diagnostic problem. However, aspiration of nonradiopaque objects is often difficult to diagnose and may require special radiographs.

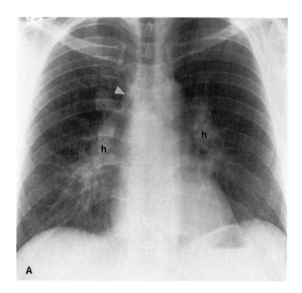

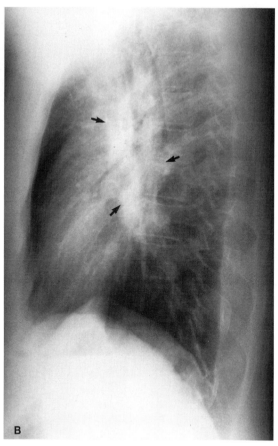

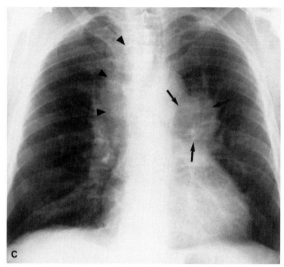

FIGURE 3-41 Chest radiographs: Examples of mediastinal and hilar adenopathy; (2) cases: (A,B) PA and lateral chest radiographs demonstrate bilateral hilar (h) and right paratracheal nodal enlargement (arrowhead). The lateral view reveals bulky adenopathy (arrows). This is a case of sarcoidosis but could easily represent lymphoma or another neoplastic process. (C) AP chest radiograph shows a large mass in the aortico-pulmonary (A-P) window (arrows). Extensive right paratracheal lymph node enlargement is present deviating the trachea to the left (arrowheads). This is a case of small-cell lung carcinoma with extensive mediastinal adenopathy. It is important to recognize abnormal mediastinal contours when evaluating chest radiographs. Any suspicious areas should be evaluated with CT.

MEDIASTINUM

Radiographically, the mediastinum is divided into numerous compartments with a differential diagnosis for any abnormal finding dependent on the compartment in which it is located. In the emergency department, it is important to examine the mediastinum for any shifting, widening, or abnormal contours that may indicate underlying hematoma, adenopathy, or mass lesion (Figure 3-41). Plain film radiographs are the initial screening tool for the mediastinum; however, most diagnostic decisions are based on CT or MRI studies. Hiatal hernias are commonly seen as a retrocardiac mediastinal mass. If an air-fluid level is present in the hernia sac, the diagnosis is assured (Figure 3-42).

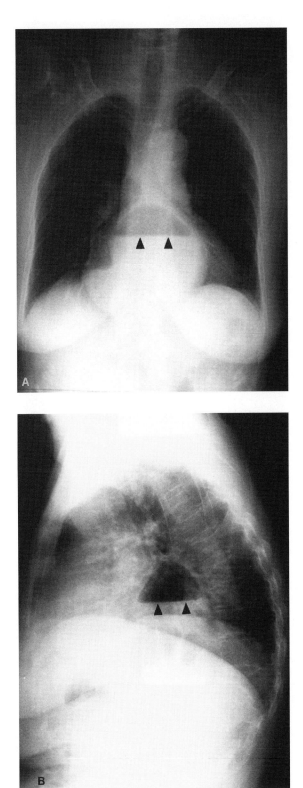

FIGURE 3-42 PA and lateral chest: Hiatal hernia: A large retrocardiac mass is visible on both the PA (A) and lateral (B) views. An air-fluid level (arrowheads) is present. These findings are diagnostic of a hiatal hernia. The air-fluid level indicates air and stomach contents contained in the hernia sac.

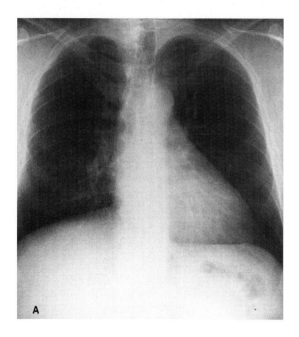
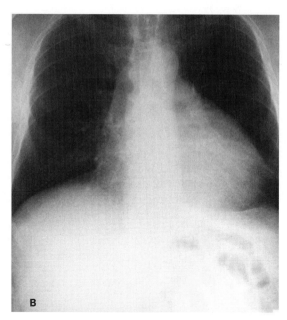

FIGURE 3-43   PA chest: Pericardial effusion: (A) PA view is normal. The cardiac silhouette is unremarkable. (B) The same patient 2 weeks later demonstrates an enlarged cardiac silhouette. Pericardial effusion was diagnosed by echocardiography.

CARDIAC SILHOUETTE

The cardiothoracic ratio is the ratio between the transverse heart measurement and the greatest internal thoracic cage measurement. Normal cardiothoracic ratio in an adult should not exceed 0.5 on standard upright PA chest radiographs.

Unfortunately, calculating the cardiothoracic ratio is subject to numerous variables that affect its accuracy. Poor inspiratory effort, supine positioning, and magnification in portable films falsely increase the heart size.

It is important to ensure that high-quality films are obtained utilizing upright PA technique with good inspiratory effort before determining that the cardiac silhouette is abnormal. This is especially true if the finding in question is subtle.

An enlarged cardiac silhouette may be produced by cardiac chamber enlargement from valvular diseases or cardiomyopathies. Fluid in the pericardial sac can also create an enlarged cardiac silhouette and is best diagnosed with echocardiography (Figure 3-43).

PLEURAL SPACES

Radiographic opacities that obscure the diaphragm and demonstrate a meniscus sign on an upright film are most commonly pleural effusions (Figure 3-44A). Aspirated fluid can be either transudative, exudative, or even bloody (Table 3-7). Patient position is important when assessing for pleural effusions. It is difficult to detect pleural fluid in the supine patient

TABLE 3-7   Differential Diagnosis of Pleural Effusion

Transduate	Exudate	Hemorrhagic
Congestive heart failure (usually right-sided effusion)	Infection	Trauma
Cirrhosis	Neoplasm	Pulmonary embolism
Renal Failure	Collagen vascular disease	
Pulmonary embolism	Pancreatitis (usually left-sided effusion)	
	Chylothorax	

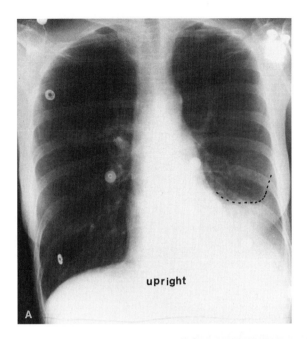

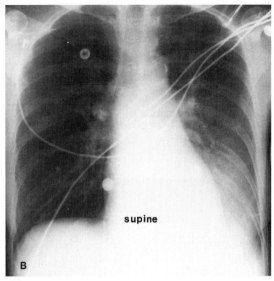

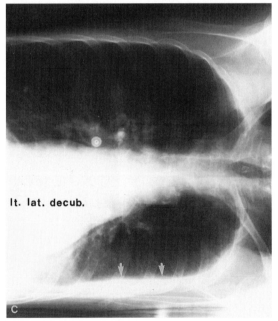

FIGURE 3-44 **PA upright, supine AP and left lateral decubitus chest: Pleural effusion:** (A) PA upright view demonstrates opacification of the left lower hemithorax. A meniscus (dashed line) indicates the pleural effusion. Effusions characteristically obscure lateral and posterior costophrenic angles. (B) Supine AP view of the same patient reveals how the left-sided effusion changes with a change in patient position. The meniscus is no longer seen. Opacification of the left lower hemithorax remains and appears more diffuse as the effusion layers posteriorly. (C) Left lateral decubitus view is obtained by positioning the patient on the left side. The pleural fluid layers along the left chest wall (arrows).

because the effusion is layered posteriorly (Figure 3-44B). Small effusions are frequently missed.

When it is clinically important to assess for the presence of an effusion or to quantitate the amount of fluid, lateral decubitus views with the involved side positioned dependently are helpful (Figure 3-44C). CT or ultrasonography may provide clinically useful information when there is a possibility of a loculated pleural fluid collection.

A subpulmonic effusion appears as an apparent elevation of the hemidiaphragm. Fluid that has accumulated beneath the lower lobe of the lung and hemidiaphragm will usually layer on lateral decubitus films (Figure 3-45).

Pleural fluid can accumulate in the interlobar fissures, simulating parenchymal lesions. These pseudo-tumors are easily identified in the fissures on radiographs (Figure 3-46). Pseudo-tumors characteristically resolve rapidly with therapy. This further helps to distinguish them from parenchymal masses.

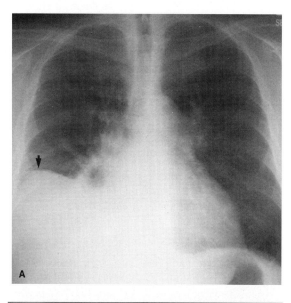

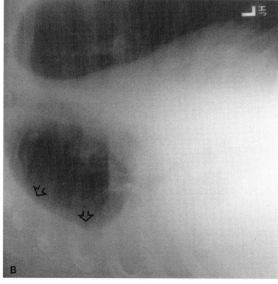

FIGURE 3-45 **PA and right lateral decubitus chest: Subpulmonic effusion:** (A) PA view demonstrates apparent elevation of the right hemidiaphragm. The peak of the right diaphragm is shifted laterally suggesting a subpulmonic effusion (arrow). (B) Right lateral decubitus view confirms the presence of an effusion as a large amount of fluid layers dependently (open arrows).

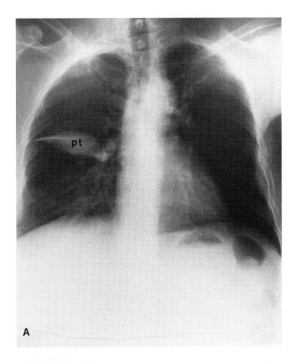

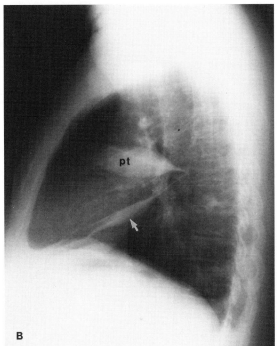

FIGURE 3-46 **PA and lateral chest: Pseudotumor:** Both PA (A) and lateral views (B) demonstrate an opacity simulating a mass in the minor fissure. This pseudotumor (pt) represents fluid that has accumulated in the fissure. A small amount of fluid also has accumulated in the right major fissure (arrow). Pseudotumors characteristically resolve quickly.

TABLE 3-8   Differential Diagnosis
             of Pneumothorax

1. Spontaneous
2. Trauma
3. Secondary to preexisting disease
   Asthma
   Emphysema
   Cystic fibrosis
   Neoplasm
   Ruptured bleb or bullae
4. Pulmonary infection
   Coccidioidomycosis
   Acute pneumonia
5. Iatrogenic
   Central line insertion
   Thoracentesis

Pleural thickening may be difficult to distinguish from a pleural effusion. Blunting of the costophrenic angle and a lack of appropriate fluid layering on lateral decubitus views are clues to the possibility of pleural thickening. Common etiologies of pleural thickening include diseases secondary to asbestos exposure, previous infection, or trauma are common etiologies. Pleural tumors, although uncommon, may present with similar findings and appear somewhat more lobulated and irregular. CT is helpful in differentiating pleural fluid from pleural thickening or pleural tumor.

PNEUMOTHORAX

Pneumothorax is usually associated with rib fractures in a patient with a history of trauma. However, numerous other etiologies exist (Table 3-8). Radiographic detection of a pneumothorax depends on the amount of air within the pleural cavity as well as the patient's position. With moderate to large intrathoracic air collections there is usually no difficulty in detection (Figure 3-47). However, when the patient is supine or the amount of intrapleural air is small, pneumothoraces are frequently missed. The usual screening examination consists of PA and lateral chest radiographs. When these views are normal and the suspicion for a pneumothorax remains high, upright PA expiratory views may demonstrate small pneumothoraces (Figure 3-48). This is because small pneumothoraces are more readily apparent when the volume of the hemithorax is reduced. In the supine patient, a deep sulcus sign is evidence of

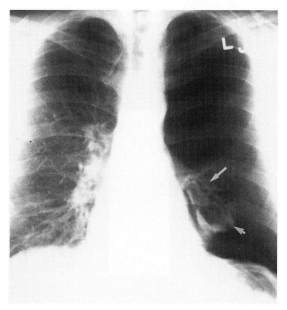

FIGURE 3-47   **PA chest: Pneumothorax:** The left hemithorax is hyperlucent due to a large pneumothorax. The collapsed lung is indicated by the arrows. It is important to evaluate the mediastinum for any shift, an indication of a tension pneumothorax. This is a case of a simple pneumothorax because the mediastinum is normal.

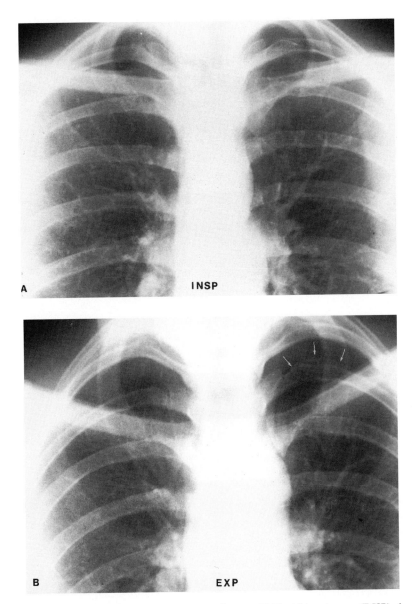

A INSP

B EXP

FIGURE 3-48 **Detail inspiratory/expiratory views: Pneumothorax:** (A) Detail inspiratory (INSP) view of upper chest is normal. (B) Repeat examination in expiration (EXP) reveals a small left apical pneumothorax (arrows). Expiratory technique reduces the chest volume accentuating any pulmonary air leaks.

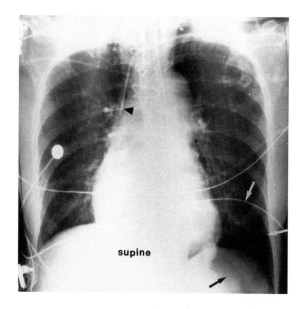

supine

←

FIGURE 3-49   **Supine AP chest: Basilar pneumothorax:** Portable AP view obtained after a left subclavian central venous catheter was inserted (arrowhead). The radiograph demonstrates a left basilar lucency representing a pneumothorax (arrows).

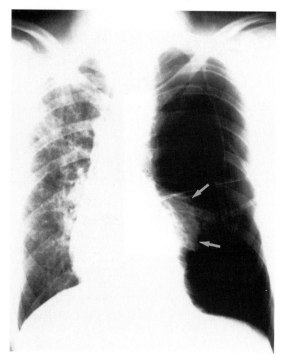

→

FIGURE 3-50   **PA chest: Tension pneumothorax:** The left hemithorax is hyperlucent and the collapsed lung, indicating a pneumothorax, is easily identified (arrows). It is extremely important not to miss the contralateral mediastinal shift indicating a tension pneumothorax.

a pneumothorax. This sign consists of a basilar lucency due to air accumulating inferiorly in the costophrenic sulcus (Figure 3-49). Estimation of pneumothorax size is difficult and often inaccurate. The clinical question should be: Does this patient require a chest tube to re-expand the lung? If, on upright chest radiograph, the pneumothorax measures 3 cm at the lateral chest wall, or 4 cm at the apex, or the patient is symptomatic, then a chest tube will most likely need to be inserted. Tension pneumothorax results from a progressive accumulation of air within the pleural space, with subsequent displacement of the mediastinal structures to the contralateral side (Figure 3-50). This usually results in severe respiratory compromise and vascular insufficiency. It is a true emergency requiring immediate treatment.

A combination of fluid and air within the thoracic cavity (hydropneumothorax) demonstrates a characteristic air-fluid level without a meniscus (Figure 3-51). The absence of a meniscus distinguishes a hydropneumothorax from a simple pleural effusion. Skin folds may cause some diagnostic confusion, and careful attention to the characteristic appearance of the skin fold is necessary. Pneumothoraces demonstrate total absence of parenchymal markings or vascular structures lateral to the lung margin. Additionally, the lung visceral pleura has a distinct white line (Figure 3-51). Skin folds, however, do not have a distinct white line but demonstrate a line that is sharply defined on one side but fades away toward the other side (Figure 3-52A). This finding represents differences in density between the skin and trapped air. Frequently, it is possible to identify lung markings lateral to the skin fold. If in doubt, a repeat upright expiratory view should clarify the situation.

Confusing the medial border of the scapula for the visceral pleural line of a collapsed lung is another pneumothorax imitator (Figure 3-52B).

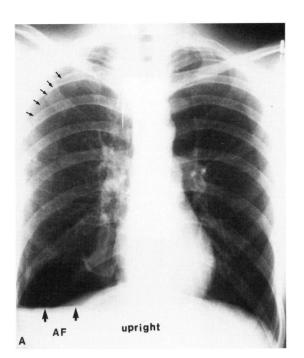
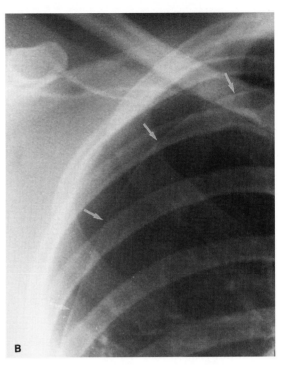

FIGURE 3-51   PA chest and right upper lobe detail view: Hydropneumothorax: (A) The upright projection demonstrates a small right apical pneumothorax (small arrows). A larger basilar pneumothorax with an air-fluid level (AF) also is present (large arrows). An important diagnostic key is the absence of a fluid meniscus. A pulmonary air leak combined with pleural fluid leads directly to a diagnosis of a hydropneumothorax. This should not be confused with simple pleural effusion. (B) Detail view of the right apex demonstrates the white visceral line of the collapsed lung (arrows).

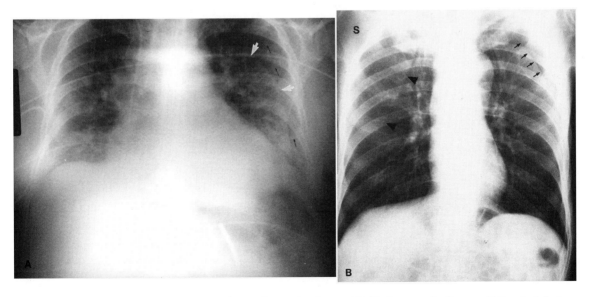

FIGURE 3-52   AP chest, different patients: Pneumothorax simulators: (A) AP view reveals a line paralleling the left chest wall (large arrows). This is a skin fold and not a pneumothorax. The white visceral line is absent and there are distal lung markings (small arrows). (B) AP view demonstrates two different pneumothorax simulators. A small skin fold is present in the left apex (arrows). The medial scapular (S) border (arrowheads) can sometimes be mistaken for a pneumothorax. If there is clinical confusion regarding a potential pneumothorax vs. an artifact, repeat the film. If possible, obtain an upright film in full respiratory expiration.

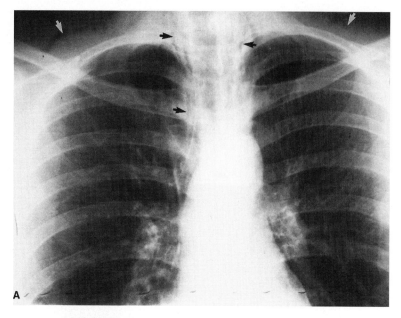

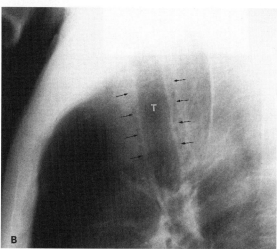

FIGURE 3-53   **Detail AP and lateral chest: Pneumomediastinum:** (A) Detail AP view of the superior mediastinum and upper chest demonstrates air outlining the airway (black arrows). Air from this pneumomediastinum also has dissected into the base of the neck (white arrows). (B) The lateral projection further illustrates the air (arrows), which outlines the trachea (T).

PNEUMOMEDIASTINUM

Pneumomediastinum is the presence of air within the mediastinum. The mechanism is an increase in intraalveolar pressure with subsequent alveolar rupture. The air then tracks along the bronchovascular bundle and may even result in a pneumothorax.

Pneumomediastinum is recognized as a lucency within the mediastinum adjacent to such structures as the main pulmonary artery, aorta, and trachea (Figure 3-53). The most common radiographic find-ing of pneumomediastinum is air outlining the left heart border (Figure 3-54). Nontraumatic causes of pneumomediastinum include strenuous exercise, childbirth, asthma, or drug use, such as smoking crack cocaine or marijuana.

Tears in either the esophagus or tracheobronchial tree are serious disorders presenting with pneumo-mediastinum. Bacterial mediastinitis is a rare cause. Air within the mediastinum may enter the neck and cause cervical subcutaneous emphysema or dissect below the diaphragm into the retroperitoneal space.

ESOPHAGEAL PERFORATION

Blunt or penetrating chest trauma can result in esophageal perforation. Severe vomiting can also result in a spectrum of esophageal injury. Mallory-Weiss syndrome is the result of vomiting that tears only the esophageal mucosa. These patients usually have upper gastrointestinal bleeding.

Boerhaave's syndrome is the severe sequelae of prolonged vomiting. Esophageal perforation occurs causing severe back, chest, or epigastric pain. In these cases, chest radiographs usually demonstrate pneumomediastinum and a left pleural effusion or hydropneumothorax.

ESOPHAGEAL FOREIGN BODY

Young children will swallow almost anything solid or liquid. They are often brought to the emergency department to determine the position of a suspected swallowed foreign body. If an abdominal film does not demonstrate the suspected object, then radiographs of the chest should be performed. Coins are common offenders, and these usually lodge at the level of the thoracic inlet (Figure 3-55). If clinical suspicion is high, and no radiopaque foreign body is identified on plain films, a barium swallow can exclude the presence of a nonradiopaque object lodged in the esophagus.

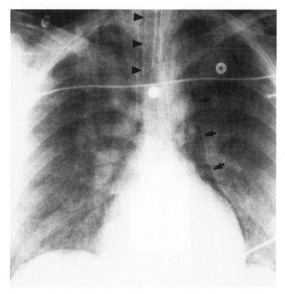

FIGURE 3-54 **PA chest: Pneumomediastinum:** PA view reveals an endotracheal tube (arrowheads) projecting into the trachea. Air outlines the left heart border, diagnostic of a pneumomediastinum.

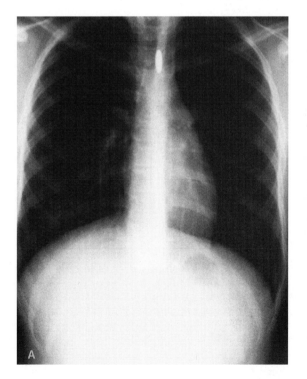
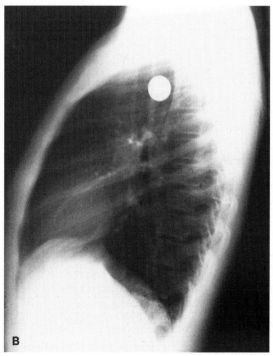

FIGURE 3-55 **PA and lateral chest: Swallowed foreign body:** PA and lateral views (A and B) reveal a coin lodged in the esophagus at the level of the thoracic inlet. The orientation of the coin is typical of an esophageal foreign body. The airway is not compromised.

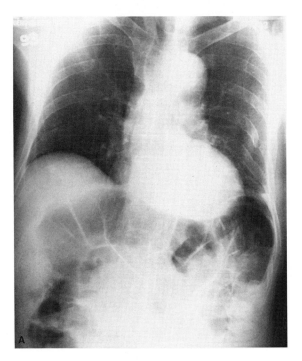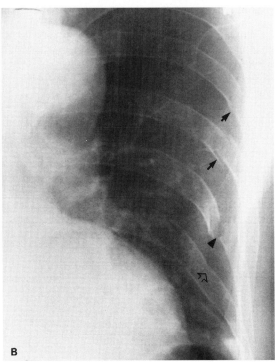

FIGURE 3-56 **AP chest with left rib detail: Multiple rib fractures:** (A) AP view demonstrates numerous left-side rib fractures. This view is important to exclude a pneumothorax or pulmonary contusion. (B) The rib detail projection illustrates the many appearances of rib fractures. Some are nondisplaced (arrows), some are displaced fractures (arrowhead), whereas others are only minimal cortical angulations (open arrow).

RIB FRACTURES

Thoracic cage trauma can result in rib fractures. The majority of rib fractures occur posteriorly, usually involving the 4th through 9th ribs (Figure 3-56). Fractures involving upper ribs have a higher morbidity due to the increased incidence of associated injury to the aorta and great vessels. Fractures of the lower ribs may be obscured by abdominal contents and are associated with trauma to abdominal organs, particularly the liver, spleen, and kidneys.

In these cases, it is important to obtain PA and lateral chest radiographs to exclude associated intrathoracic trauma, such as pulmonary contusion or pneumothorax. Subcutaneous emphysema of the chest wall is an indirect sign of rib fracture.

A flail chest represents segmental fractures of three or more ribs. Patients usually present with marked respiratory compromise and have a high probability of underlying pulmonary parenchymal injury. Observation of the thorax may demonstrate paradoxical chest wall motion.

Thoracic cage trauma in children usually does not cause rib fractures. When rib fractures are identified in the pediatric population, one should consider the possibility of child abuse (Figure 5-24).

PULMONARY CONTUSION

Lung contusion usually is a sequela of blunt chest wall trauma. The injured lung becomes radiographically opaque as fluid and blood leak into the tissues and alveoli. Pulmonary contusions are usually patchy and ill-defined radiographically. Characteristically, they are present on the initial examination or occur relatively quickly after the initial injury (Figure 3-57). Worsening opacification may occur up to 48 hours following the initial insult, but chest radiographs usually begin to show clearing within 72 hours. Persistent worsening outside of this time frame is usually a result of superimposed atelectasis, pneumonia, or persistent hemorrhage.

Traumatic lung cysts are seen as lucencies in the lung following trauma. Air-fluid levels may be present. As the cyst becomes organized, it may appear as a well-rounded or even oval density that takes weeks to resolve (Figure 3-58).

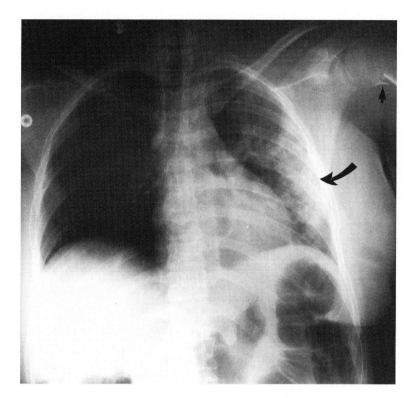

FIGURE 3-57 **AP chest: Pulmonary contusion:** A large area of consolidation in the left chest secondary to blunt thoracic trauma (curved arrow) is visible. The air-space process is a combination of alveolar and interstitial edema with hemorrhage. Note the associated proximal humeral fracture (arrow).

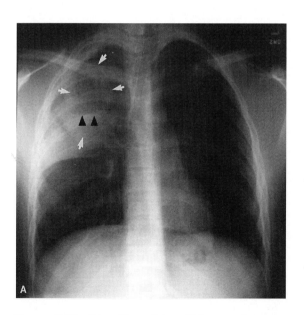
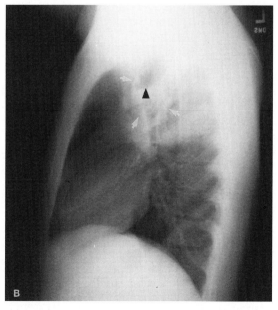

FIGURE 3-58 **PA and lateral chest: Pulmonary hematoma and laceration:** PA and lateral projections (A and B) reveal an area of consolidation in the right upper lobe secondary to blunt trauma. Contained within this hematoma is a cystic space (arrows) containing an air-fluid level (arrowheads). This traumatic lung cyst resulted from a parenchymal laceration.

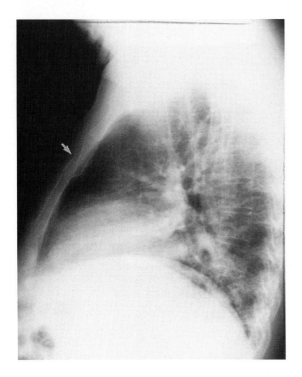

←

FIGURE 3-59 **Lateral chest: Sternal fracture:** This patient's chest hit the steering wheel during an automobile accident. A sternal fracture (arrow) occurred. These patients need to be evaluated for a possible cardiac or pulmonary contusion.

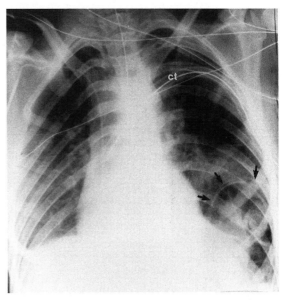

→

FIGURE 3-60 **AP chest: Ruptured diaphragm:** The initial AP view of this patient demonstrates poor definition of the left hemidiaphragm. Loops of bowel that have herniated into the chest are visible (arrows). A right CVP line, nasogastric tube, and left chest tube (CT) are present. A ruptured diaphragm is frequently missed on initial presentation. A high index of suspicion should be maintained anytime there is an abnormal contour of the hemidiaphragm.

STERNAL FRACTURES

Direct trauma to the sternum from a steering wheel is the usual clinical presentation for a sternal fracture (Figure 3-59). Commonly, a fracture dislocation occurs at the manubrial sternal joint. Sternal fractures are associated with fractures of the spinal column. Cardiac and pulmonary contusions are frequent complications seen with sternal injury.

DIAPHRAGM

Trauma to the lower thoracic cage or upper abdomen can result in a rent or tear in the diaphragm. This occurs more commonly on the left, as it is felt the liver affords some protection to the right dome of the diaphragm (Figure 3-60). Initial diagnosis may be difficult without obvious herniation of the stomach or abdominal contents into the thoracic cavity. Suspicion for diaphragmatic injury should be maintained anytime there is apparent elevation of the diaphragm on the initial AP chest radiograph. Associated injuries involving the liver, spleen, and retroperitoneal structures are common. Solid organ herniation on the right is even more difficult to detect than left-sided diaphragmatic herniations.

An abnormal course of the nasogastric tube into the chest cavity is the characteristic finding seen with left diaphragmatic rupture and gastric herniation. Barium studies may be of benefit in establishing the position of gastrointestinal structures when faced with an abnormal chest radiograph.

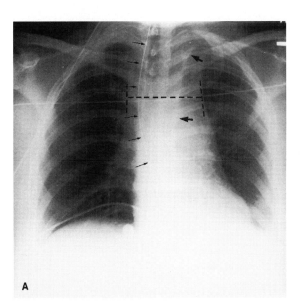
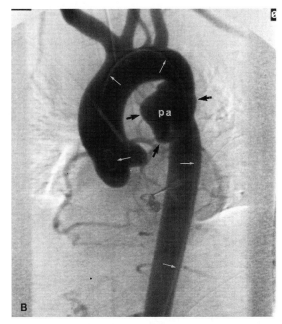

FIGURE 3-61 AP chest and aortogram: Acute traumatic aortic injury (ATAI): (A) This AP view demonstrates many of the plain-film indicators of ATAI; the superior mediastinum is widened (dashed lines), the nasogastric tube is deviated to the right (small arrows), the aortic knob is obscured, and the paraspinous stripe is widened and continues above the aortic knob (large arrows). (B) The aortogram is performed by inserting a catheter into the root of the aorta (white arrows), usually from a femoral artery approach. The traumatic pseudoaneurysm (PA) is usually located just distal to the origin of the left subclavian artery (black arrows).

ACUTE TRAUMATIC AORTIC INJURY (ATAI)

Rapid deceleration injuries can result in traumatic injury to the aorta and great vessels. ATAI usually results in immediate death. However, a small number of patients will survive to be transported to the emergency department. There are numerous plain-film indicators of ATAI (Table 3-9). Although none of these findings are specific, the key to diagnosis is the detection of a mediastinal hematoma (Figure 3-61A).

The gold standard in establishing the diagnosis is emergent thoracic aortography. The aortic tear is located, most commonly, just distal to the origin of the left subclavian artery at the aortic isthmus (Figure 3-61B). Once identified, this is a true emergency as many of these patients will succumb to this injury in a short period of time.

CT of the chest has been advocated to detect the presence of a mediastinal hematoma. This is a time-consuming procedure and should only be utilized when the patient is stable and the likelihood of injury is low. If the CT examination is positive, the patient will subsequently require aortography to confirm the diagnosis. Evaluation of the patient with suspected ATAI is included in Algorithm 3-3.

TABLE 3-9   Plain Film Findings of Acute Traumatic Aortic Injury (ATAI)

1. Superior mediastinal widening: > 8 cm
2. Obscured aortic knob or abnormal aortic contour
3. Abnormal paraspinous stripe: widened or continuing above aortic knob
4. Blood in thoracic apex: "Apical cap"
5. Abnormally widened right paratracheal stripe: > 5 mm
6. Nasogastric tube deviated to the right

ALGORITHM 3-3   **Evaluation of the Patient with Suspected Acute Traumatic Aortic Injury (ATAI)**

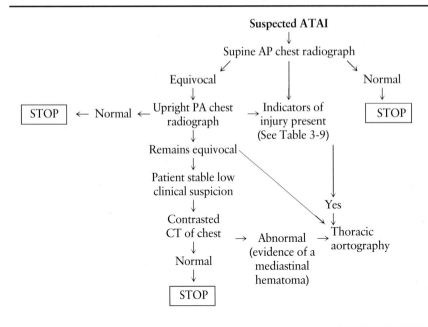

THORACIC AORTIC DISSECTION

Hypertension is the most common etiology for thoracic aortic dissections. Acutely, the patient has chest pain, which may radiate into the back. Aortic dissections are difficult to detect on chest radiographs; they can rupture and result in death. CT, MRI, thoracic aortography, and transesophageal echo are diagnostic.

CT is commonly the screening examination of choice to diagnose a dissection. It is performed using sequential bolus injections of iodinated contrast and scanning at the level of the aortic arch, aortic root, and level of the diaphragmatic aorta. CT diagnosis of a dissection includes dilatation of the aorta and, more specifically, identification of a double lumen. This double lumen represents true and false lumens separated by an intimal flap (Figure 3-62).

TUBES AND LINES

Critically ill patients often require placement of many different tubes and lines during their care.

Radiographs are used to both determine the tube or line position and to be sure there are no complications. The most commonly seen tubes and lines are endotracheal, nasogastric, central venous, and chest. Their placement and associated complications are discussed below.

Endotracheal Tube (ETT)

Management of the airway is the number one priority during patient resuscitation. The ETT is easily identified on portable AP chest films (Figure 3-63). The ETT tip should be at least 1 cm above the carina in both children and adults, and it should be no higher than the level of the suprasternal notch. Common problems with ETT placement are inserting the tube too deeply into the main stem bronchi (usually right) (Figure 3-16) or inserting it in the esophagus. A misplaced tube in the esophagus can be difficult to detect on AP supine chest radiographs as it may appear satisfactorily positioned within the trachea when it is actually in the esophagus. Check the stomach for air distention, but most importantly, pay attention to clinical clues.

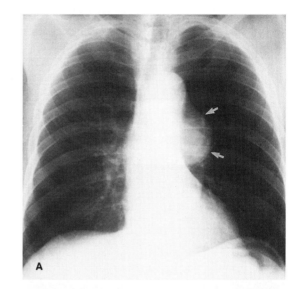

FIGURE 3-62 AP chest and CT chest: Dissecting thoracic aorta: (A) AP view reveals an abnormal contour of the descending thoracic aorta (arrows). (B) Dynamic CT with contrast at the level of the aortic arch demonstrates a flap (open arrow) indicating a dissection. (C) Dynamic CT at the level of the left atrium (la) again demonstrates the flap (open arrow) separating the true (t) from the false (f) lumen. The right ventricle (rv) and aortic root (ao) also are visible.

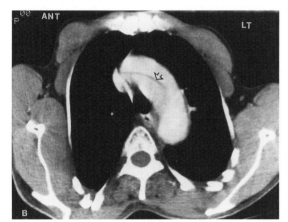

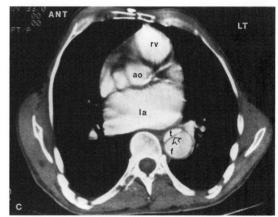

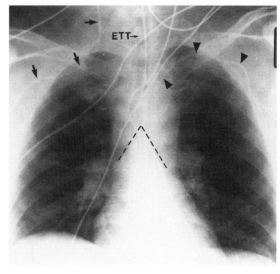

FIGURE 3-63 AP supine chest: Malpositioned right subclavian vein catheter: The right subclavian venous catheter has turned upward into the jugular vein (arrows). A second subclavian venous catheter is identified on the right (arrowheads). Numerous overlying EKG wires obscure visualization of the tip of the left central line. An endotracheal tube (ETT) projects in good position above the carina (dashed lines). No pneumothorax is seen.

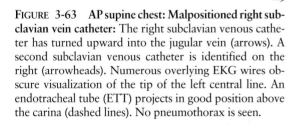

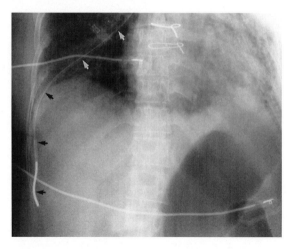

FIGURE 3-64 **Detail AP view lower chest: Feeding tube in the pleural space:** An enteric feeding tube was inserted at the bedside. Post-placement radiograph was obtained prior to initiating tube feedings. The feeding tube was inserted into the patient's airway, advanced through the right main-stem bronchus, perforated the right lung, and became lodged in the pleural space (arrows).

Nasogastric Tube (NGT)

The normal course of an NGT is through the esophagus into the stomach. The most serious potential complication that can result from placing a NGT is placing it into the tracheobronchial tree (Figures 3-64, 3-65). There also have been a few instances of patients with severe maxillofacial trauma in whom the NGT entered the calvarium.

Central Venous Lines

Insertion of a catheter into the central circulation is commonly performed by either a subclavian or internal jugular venous puncture. The tip of a correctly placed catheter should be in the superior vena cava, approximately 1 to 4 cm below the medial aspect of the right clavicle (Figure 3-66). The most common problem associated with the misplacement of subclavian catheters occurs when the tube turns cephalad into the jugular vein (Figure 3-63) or when it crosses the midline into the opposite subclavian vein (Figure 3-67). Other possible complications of central-line insertion are pneumothorax (Figure 3-49) and mediastinal hematoma.

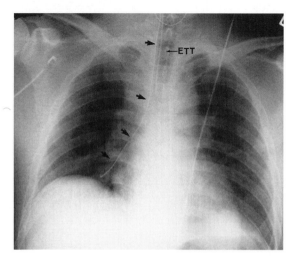

FIGURE 3-65 **AP chest: Nasogastric tube (NGT) in right main-stem bronchus:** NGT is seen in this patient's right main-stem bronchus (arrows). An endotracheal tube (ETT) projects in good position above the carina.

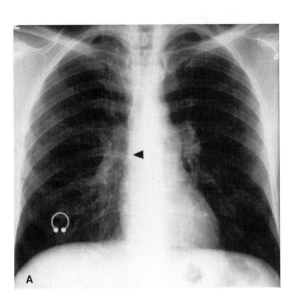

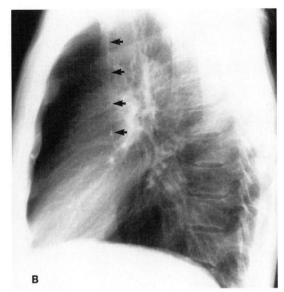

FIGURE 3-66   PA and lateral chest: Correctly positioned central venous catheter: (A) AP chest radiograph demonstrates a right-sided central line with the tip in the distal superior vena cava (SVC) (arrowhead). A nipple ring is seen on the right. (B) Lateral projection confirms correct placement of the catheter tip in the SVC (arrows). Note the normal position of the SVC on frontal and lateral projections.

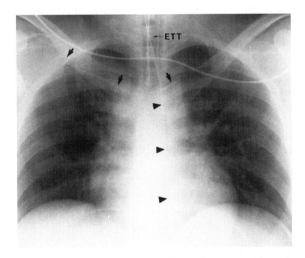

FIGURE 3-67   AP chest: Malpositioned right subclavian venous catheter: Right-sided subclavian venous catheter is seen crossing the midline into the contralateral subclavian vein (arrows). An endotracheal tube (ETT) and a nasogastric tube (arrowheads) are both in good position. No pneumothorax is seen.

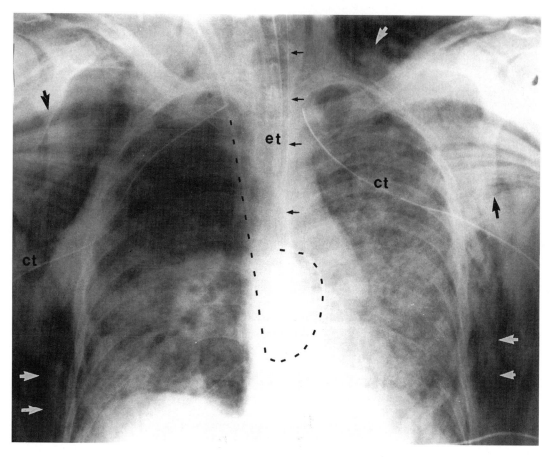

FIGURE 3-68 **AP supine chest: Subcutaneous emphysema:** This trauma patient with ARDS required high ventilator pressures to maintain oxygenation. Bilateral pneumothoraces occurred and were treated with chest tubes (ct). The endotracheal tube (et) appears to be in good position. The Swan-Ganz catheter (dashed line) and nasogastric tube (small arrows) are visible. Bilateral parenchymal opacities of ARDS are present. No definite remaining pneumothorax is visible. However, there is extensive bilateral subcutaneous emphysema (large arrows) dissecting laterally into the chest walls, the pectoralis muscles, and cephalad into the neck.

Chest Tubes

Most chest tubes inserted in the emergency department are to evacuate a pneumothorax. Post-placement chest radiographs should demonstrate that all the side holes of the chest tube are in the chest cavity, the tube is not kinked and the pneumothorax is reducing (Figure 3-68).

Chapter 3 Chest Pearls _____

1. Portable AP radiographs *magnify* intrathoracic structures.
2. Epiglottitis is a medical emergency. A physician experienced in pediatric airway management should be in attendance with the child.
3. An upper-lobe air-space process may be reactivation tuberculosis.
4. Patients in early CHF may present to the emergency department with a complaint of coughing. Their clinical exam is often normal. Careful inspection of their chest radiographs is necessary to accurately make the diagnosis of early CHF.
5. Many patients with pulmonary emboli have normal chest radiographs.
6. Common diseases such as pneumonia or CHF present atypically in patients with COPD.
7. Persistent air-space disease following antibiotic therapy suggests an obstructive process.

Consider the possibility of an endobronchial foreign body in a child and bronchogenic carcinoma in an adult.

8. Don't forget that a pericardial effusion mimics an enlarged heart. Check for signs of impaired venous return.

9. Don't mistake skin folds for a pneumothorax.

10. Assess the position of the mediastinum in every patient with a pneumothorax to exclude a tension pneumothorax.

11. A small pneumothorax is often missed on standard PA and lateral chest films. Consider an upright PA expiratory chest radiograph.

12. Patients with acute pneumonia may not develop radiographic findings for up to 12 hours after the onset of symptoms.

13. Consider the possibility of tuberculosis in any homeless, immunocompromised or institutionalized patient who presents with pneumonia.

14. Prior chest radiographs for comparison purposes are a clinician's best friend.

4

Abdomen, Urinary Tract, and Pelvis

OVERVIEW

Numerous studies have shown that in the absence of either severe abdominal pain or clinical concern for pneumoperitoneum or intestinal obstruction, plain films are rarely useful in the clinical management of patients with abdominal symptoms. Abdominal radiographs have largely been replaced by ultrasonography and computed tomography.

TECHNIQUES

Plain Films

Plain films are most effective detecting either bowel obstruction or pneumoperitoneum. An upright abdominal examination combined with a supine view is necessary to identify small amounts of free intraperitoneal air or air-fluid levels. If the

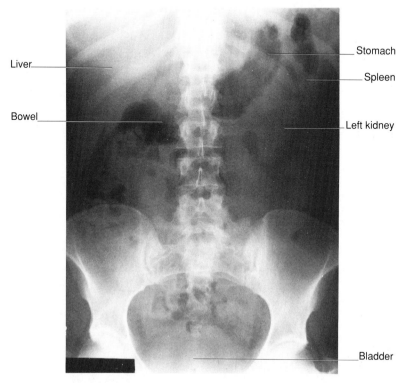

FIGURE 4-1 Supine abdominal radiograph: Normal anatomy

patient is too ill to undergo an upright examination, a left lateral decubitus view can be substituted. A normal supine view is shown in Figure 4-1.

Ultrasonography

Ultrasonography is often used to evaluate abdominal and pelvic structures in patients who come to the emergency department with acute pain. The majority of the studies ordered are the following: right upper quadrant ultrasound to assess the gallbladder and biliary structures, renal ultrasound to exclude hydronephrosis, and pelvic ultrasound to exclude ectopic pregnancy (Table 4-1).

Nuclear Medicine

A radionuclide hepatobiliary scan is frequently ordered in a patient with right upper quadrant pain to assess patency of the cystic duct. Testicular scans are infrequently ordered but are important in differentiating missed testicular torsion from acute epididymitis.

Computed Tomography

CT is the imaging study of choice for evaluating hemodynamically stable trauma victims. CT is also useful when evaluating a patient suspected of having an abdominal aortic aneurysm.

Oral Contrast Agents

Plain-film and fluoroscopic evaluation of the gastrointestinal tract can be done with either water-soluble or barium-contrast agents. These can be used to evaluate patients for suspected perforation or intestinal obstruction. Infrequently, contrast agents are used to clarify organ position, particularly the stomach, in a patient suspected of having a diaphragmatic hernia.

Intravenous Urogram (IVU)

IVUs, also known as intravenous pyelograms (IVPs) are ordered to evaluate the urinary tract in patients with suspected stone disease and obstruction.

TABLE 4-1   Commonly Requested Ultrasound Exams

Exam	Reasons to order	Areas examined	Patient Preparation
Right Upper Quadrant (RUQ)	R/O cholelithiasis, biliary obstruction	Liver, biliary tree, gallbladder and right kidney	NPO at least 4 hours prior to exam
Pelvic ultrasound			
Transabdominal	R/O ectopic pregnancy or adnexal mass, pelvic pain	Uterus and adnexa	Bladder **must** be full. Patient should drink 32 oz of H_2O 1 hour prior to exam or have a Foley catheter inserted
Endovaginal	Same as above. Detects intrauterine gestations earlier than transabdominal exam	Uterus and adnexa	None Note: it is often advantageous to begin with a transabdominal pelvic ultrasound in which case the patient's bladder must be full
Renal	R/O hydronephrosis	Kidneys and bladder	None
Abdominal	Same as RUQ, more of a screening exam	Same as RUQ but also examines left kidney and spleen	NPO at least 4 hours prior to exam
Aorta	R/O abdominal aortic aneurysm	Abdominal aorta	None
Lower extremity venous Doppler	R/O DVT	Lower extremity veins	None
Right Lower Quadrant	R/O appendicitis	Area of patient's pain in an attempt to identify a diseased appendix	None

ALGORITHM 4-1   Evaluation of Abdominal Trauma

DPL = Diagnostic peritoneal lavage
CECT = Contrast-enhanced computed tomography

ABDOMINAL EVALUATION

Abdominal/Pelvic Traumatic Emergencies

Plain films are not very useful for evaluating soft-tissue injuries in the acutely traumatized patient. They are insensitive and time consuming. The chief methods for evaluating the traumatized patient's abdomen are diagnostic peritoneal lavage (DPL) and contrast-enhanced CT (CECT) (Algorithm 4-1).

DPL is advocated because it can be performed quickly in the trauma room and is more sensitive than CECT in the detection of bowel injuries. CECT is useful for identifying hemoperitoneum as well as evaluating injury to individual organs. CECT is also more sensitive than DPL in evaluating the retroperitoneum. It is important to remember that CECT is indicated only in patients who are hemodynamically stable. Unstable patients need either a DPL or emergent surgery.

Liver, spleen, and renal injuries are easily identified with contrast-enhanced CT (Figure 4-2). Findings range from contusion to frank organ fracture. The spleen is the most commonly traumatized solid organ; the liver and kidneys are the next most commonly injured. CT examination is limited in the detection of bowel injuries.

Injury to the urinary tract is common particularly in patients with pelvic fractures. Bladder catheterization is extremely important in the treatment of the severely traumatized patient. However, certain situations preclude the immediate placement of a urethral Foley. A retrograde urethrogram may need to be performed to exclude urethral injury prior to insertion of a Foley catheter if there is blood at the urethral meatus or a high-rising prostate on rectal exam (Figure 4-3). After evaluation of the urethra, the integrity of the bladder is commonly in question and a cystogram needs to be performed.

Bladder rupture can be divided into intra- or extra-peritoneal types. Intraperitoneal rupture occurs from a tear in the dome of the bladder and is diagnosed by contrast spillage into the colonic gutters and intraperitoneal space.

Extraperitoneal rupture is much more common than the intraperitoneal type and is diagnosed on cystography by extravasation of contrast into the extraperitoneal spaces (Figure 4-4). Cystography may also show an intact bladder that has been displaced by a large pelvic hematoma (Figure 4-5).

Nontraumatic Abdominal Emergencies

On plain-film radiographs, outlines of the liver, spleen, kidneys, and bladder should be assessed for their presence, size, position, and configuration. The liver appears as a homogenous right upper quadrant density of variable size. The normal liver should measure less than 15 cm in the mid-clavicular line. However, a congenital variant, such as a Reidel's lobe or flattening of the hemidiaphragms from obstructive lung disease, can simulate hepatomegaly.

The spleen is a small structure, approximately the size of a kidney, in the lateral aspect of the left upper quadrant beneath the hemidiaphragm. It is located

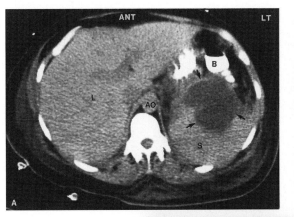

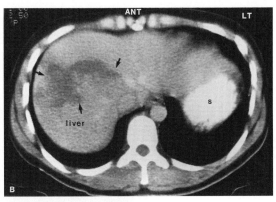

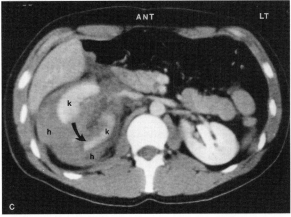

FIGURE 4-2   Abdominal CT: Blunt abdominal trauma, (3) cases: (A) A large, low attenuation, subacute hematoma (arrows) is present in the spleen (s). Contrast is visible in adjacent bowel (B). The liver (L) and aorta (AO) are normal. (B) A low attenuation laceration with irregular margins is present in the right lobe of the liver (arrows). Orally administered contrast is present in the stomach (S). (C) The right kidney (k) is bivalved by a large midpole laceration (curved arrow). A large perirenal hematoma (h) is present.

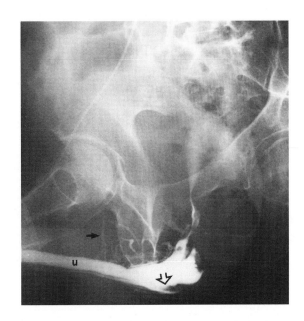

FIGURE 4-3   Retrograde urethrogram: Urethral injury: Contrast injected into the urethra (u) is extravasating into the adjacent tissues through a small laceration (open arrow). Contrast is also opacifying the adjacent venous plexus (arrow).

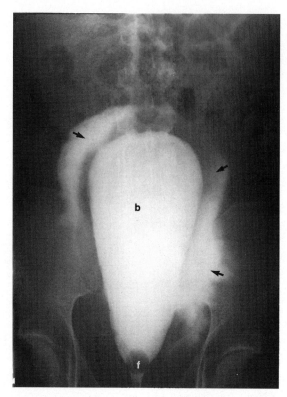

FIGURE 4-4 **Cystogram: Extraperitoneal bladder rupture:** The bladder (b) is well opacified with contrast instilled through the patient's Foley catheter (f). Extravasating contrast is identified outlining the bladder (arrows). This contrast is contained in the perivesical space and is prevented from extending further cephalad by the intact pelvic peritoneum.

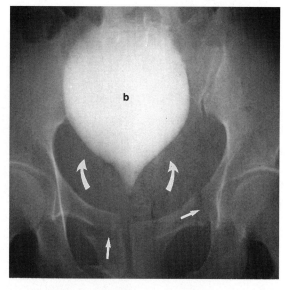

FIGURE 4-5 **Cystogram: Pelvic hematoma:** The bladder (b) is elevated and deformed by a large pelvic hematoma (curved arrows). Fractures of the anterior arch of the pelvis are also present (arrows).

lateral to the gastric bubble. Accurate splenic measurement is difficult on plain film, but gross splenomegaly is easily identified (Figure 4-6).

The kidneys are bilateral, symmetric structures with the right kidney being somewhat lower than the left due to the position of the liver. Normal adult kidneys average between three and four lumbar vertebral bodies in length.

The bladder may be outlined by fat in the pelvic midline. Bladder outlet obstruction can result in marked bladder distention (Figure 4-7).

One of the most common uses for plain films of the abdomen is to assess the bowel gas pattern. The small bowel is identified by locating the valvulae conniventes. These are parallel lines that extend across the bowel diameter. The large bowel is identified by irregular haustral lines that do not extend across the diameter of the bowel. Additionally, the large bowel is located more peripherally within the abdomen. It is normal to have an air-fluid level within the patient's stomach on an upright or decubitus examination. Other nonpathologic air-fluid levels are seen in the proximal small bowel. These are common in patients who consume carbonated beverages.

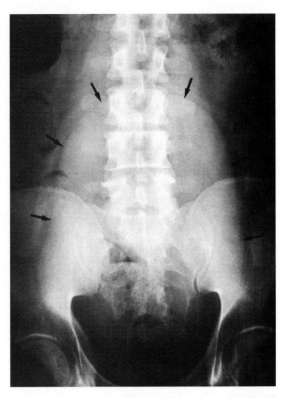

FIGURE 4-7 **Supine abdominal radiograph: Bladder distention:** Arrows outline a large soft-tissue mass in the pelvis and lower abdomen. The origin of the mass is in the pelvis and was proven to be a greatly distended bladder.

Intra-abdominal calcifications can be numerous. Some of these are incidental findings and must be differentiated from pathologic entities. The more common calcifications identified include: (1) calcified gallstones (Figure 4-8); (2) calcified mesenteric nodes, usually the sequela of prior granulomatous disease such as histoplasmosis or tuberculosis (Figure 4-25); (3) appendicolith (Figure 4-9); (4) phlebolith, which are calcified venous thrombi with central lucencies (Figure 4-10); (5) pancreatic calcifications, usually the sequela of chronic pancreatitis (Figure 4-11); (6) urinary tract stones, seen anywhere from the kidneys through the ureters into the bladder (Figure 4-12); and (7) tumors, classically calcifications of benign uterine fibroids (Figure 4-13).

All bones visible on an abdominal radiograph should be examined for fractures or destructive lesions.

The properitoneal fat line or flank stripe should be identified. It appears as a longitudinal fat lucency located along the lateral aspects of the abdominal wall (Figure 4-14). It is not present in everyone, especially thin elderly patients. Intra-abdominal fluid (Figure 4-15) or adjacent inflammatory disease such as appendicitis can obliterate the flank stripe.

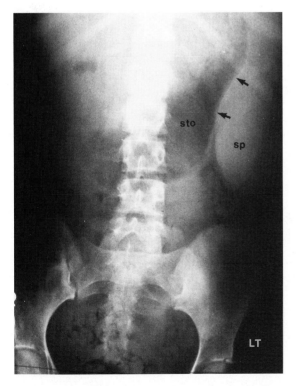

FIGURE 4-6 **Supine abdominal radiograph: Splenomegaly:** The spleen (sp) is markedly enlarged and compressing the lateral stomach (sto) margin (arrows). The spleen tip is well below the costal margin.

Text continued on page 106.

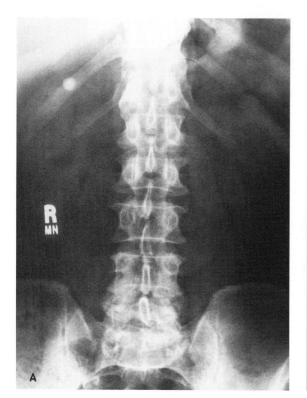

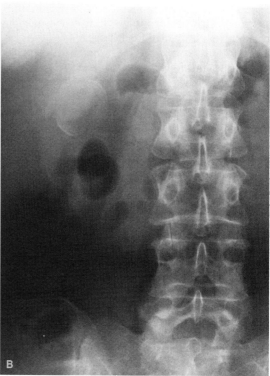

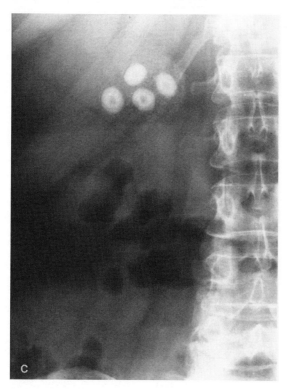

FIGURE 4-8   **Plain-film radiographs: Gallstones:** Calcified gallstones are easily identified on plain films and may be single or multiple. Depending on their composition, they can be densely calcified (A), rim calcified (B), or laminated in their appearance (C).

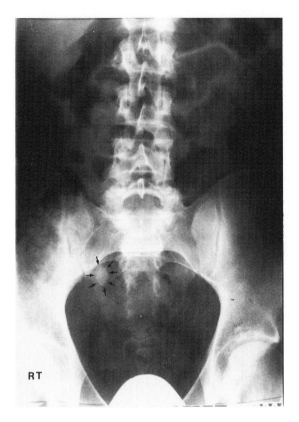

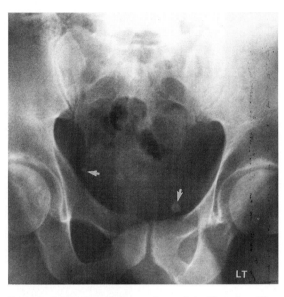

FIGURE 4-10 **Coned-down view pelvis: Vascular phleboliths:** Two calcific densities are seen in the pelvis (arrows). The larger density on the left has a central lucency diagnostic of a phlebolith. Phleboliths can vary in size and number. In some instances, it may be important to exclude a distal ureteral stone.

FIGURE 4-9 **Supine abdominal radiograph: Appendicolith:** Arrows outline a calcified appendicolith or fecalith in the right lower quadrant (RLQ). This finding in a patient with (RLQ) pain is highly suspicious for acute appendicitis.

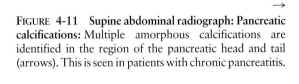

FIGURE 4-11 **Supine abdominal radiograph: Pancreatic calcifications:** Multiple amorphous calcifications are identified in the region of the pancreatic head and tail (arrows). This is seen in patients with chronic pancreatitis.

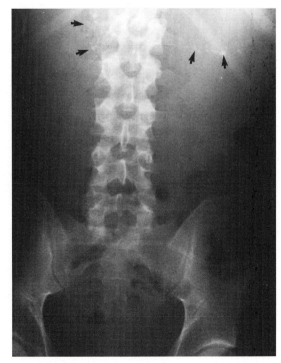

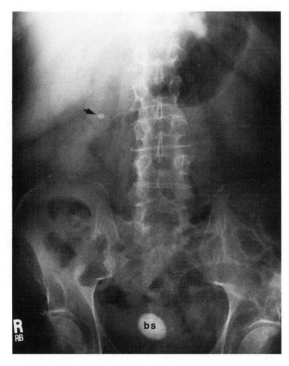

FIGURE 4-12   **Supine abdominal radiograph: Urinary tract stones:** A small calcified right renal stone (arrow) is visible in this patient who also has a large bladder stone (bs).

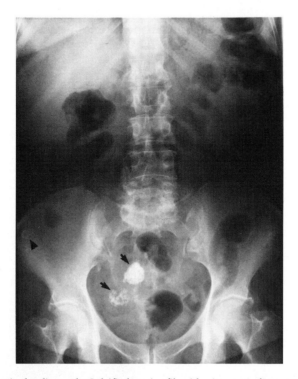

FIGURE 4-13   **Supine abdominal radiograph: Calcified uterine fibroids:** Arrows indicate two calcified uterine fibroids. A small injection granuloma is present in the right buttock (arrowhead). This represents the sequela of a prior intramuscular injection.

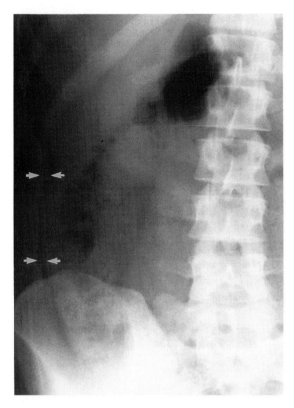

FIGURE 4-14 **Coned-down plain film: Normal properitoneal fat line:** Arrows indicate the properitoneal fat in the lateral abdominal wall. Intra-abdominal fluid, such as ascites or hemorrhage, as well as an intra-abdominal inflammatory process can obscure this fat line.

→

FIGURE 4-15 **Supine AP abdomen: Ascites:** Distal portion of a nasogastric tube is visible in the stomach (arrows). The abdomen has a diffuse hazy or "ground glass" appearance. The flank stripe is obscured. These findings are characteristic of ascites. An additional film finding of ascites is elevation of the diaphragm because of the increase in abdominal volume. Intra-abdominal fluid may be missed on plain radiographs but is visible with either ultrasound or CT. As in this case, liver disease is the most common cause of ascites.

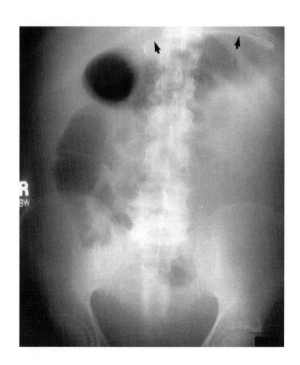

TABLE 4-2   Evaluation of Abdominal Plain Films

Structure	Findings	Differential Diagnosis
Bowel Gas	Dilated small bowel (> 3 cm)	Small-bowel obstruction (Table 4-5)
		Intestinal ileus
		Sentinel loop
	Dilated large bowel (> 5 cm)	Colonic volvulus
		Colonic obstruction—exclude neoplasm
	Paucity or absent bowel gas	Obstructed fluid-filled bowel loops
		Prolonged vomiting
Abnormal air collections	Bowel	(See above)
	Extraluminal	Pneumoperitoneum (Table 4-4)
		Abscess
		Portal venous gas
		Biliary air
Calcifications	Pathologic	Renal stones
		Appendicolith
		Gallstones
		Vascular-abdominal aortic aneurysm
	Nonpathologic	Mesenteric nodes
		Uterine fibroids
		Vascular phleboliths
Organ outlines	Liver	Size, position, configuration, and presence
	Spleen	
	Kidneys	
Properitoneal "Flank" stripe	Absent	Suspect intraperitoneal fluid or infection
Bones	Exclude fractures/lesions	
Lung bases	Exclude atelectasis, pneumonia or mass	

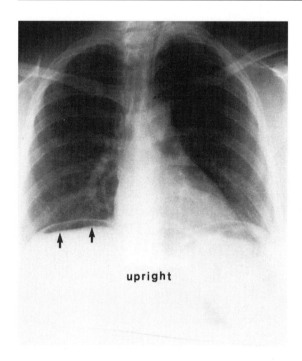

upright

FIGURE 4-16   **Upright chest radiograph: Pneumoperitoneum:** Free intra-abdominal air is visible beneath the right hemidiaphragm (arrows).

Table 4-2 lists the structures that need to be evaluated on abdominal radiographs and includes a limited differential diagnosis of abnormal findings.

Pneumoperitoneum   Small bubbles (1 to 2 mm) of free intraperitoneal air can be identified on upright abdominal examinations. This free air will accumulate beneath the right hemidiaphragm (Figure 4-16). Free air is less common beneath the left hemidiaphragm due to the phrenicocolic ligament. In patients who cannot stand, obtaining a left lateral decubitus view with the right side up will demonstrate pneumoperitoneum or free air accumulating over the right lobe of the liver (Figure 4-17). Rupture of a hollow viscus is probably the most common cause of pneumoperitoneum, although intra-abdominal abscesses or trauma can result in free intraperitoneal air (Table 4-3).

Supine examinations are limited in detecting small amounts of free air. However, large amounts of free air may present as the ability to visualize both sides of the bowel wall. This is know as Rigler's sign (Figure 4-18). Careful attention should be paid to unusual-appearing lucencies on supine views, particularly when these lucencies do not appear to be associated with bowel loops.

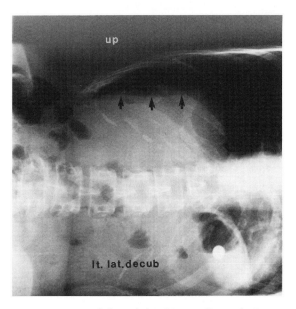

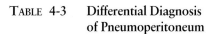

FIGURE 4-17 **Left lateral decubitus radiograph: Pneumoperitoneum:** Free intraperitoneal air is accumulating over the liver (arrows). This is a very useful examination to obtain anytime the patient cannot undergo an upright study.

Colonic interposition occurs when the colon, particularly the hepatic flexure, becomes superimposed between the liver and right hemidiaphragm (Figure 4-19). Be careful not to confuse colonic air with pneumoperitoneum.

TABLE 4-3   **Differential Diagnosis of Pneumoperitoneum**

Perforated viscus
  peptic ulcer
  diverticulitis
  appendicitis
  toxic megacolon
  intestinal infarction
Neoplasm
Iatrogenic
  recent surgery including laparoscopic procedures

Portal Venous Air Mesentery ischemia can result in gangrenous bowel. As the bowel becomes necrotic, air can dissect into the mesenteric veins. This air is then returned to the liver via the portal venous system. The air accumulates in the liver and appears as irregularly shaped lucencies in the liver periphery (Figure 4-20). Portal venous air is a grave prognostic indicator. Infants with necrotizing enterocolitis can also have portal venous gas.

Biliary Air Air within the biliary tree is seen in patients who have had prior surgery, particularly common duct diversions such as a choledochojejunostomy. Included in the differential diagnosis of biliary air are gallstone ileus, trauma, or cholangitis (Figure 4-21).

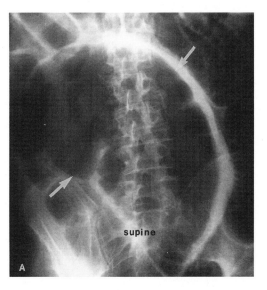

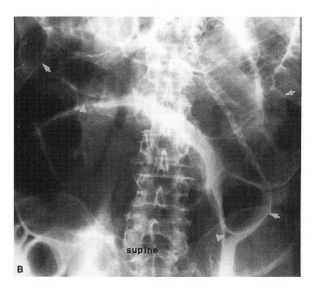

FIGURE 4-18 **Supine abdominal radiographs: Cecal volvulus with perforation:** (A) Greatly dilated colon (arrows) is visible in the mid abdomen. Loops of dilated small bowel are also present and are compatible with a diagnosis of obstruction. (B) Same patient 12 hours later. Again noted are loops of dilated large and small bowel. Free intraperitoneal air in combination with intestinal gas allows clear visualization of both sides of the bowel wall (arrows). Small pockets of free air are also visible (arrowheads). This is a case of surgically proven cecal volvulus with perforation.

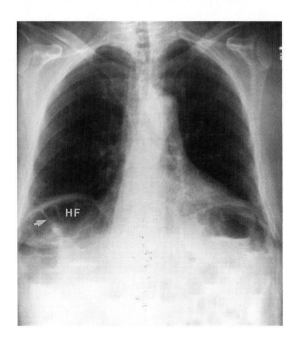

←

FIGURE 4-19 **Upright chest radiograph: Colonic interposition:** The hepatic flexure (HF) is situated beneath the right hemidiaphragm. Note the haustral markings indicating this is bowel (arrow). This should not be confused with free intraperitoneal air. If in doubt, a left lateral decubitus film would be beneficial.

Abdominal/pelvic Abscess   Intra-abdominal or pelvic infection can present as diffuse peritonitis or abscess of any organ. The most specific finding on plain films is the identification of a localized area of extralumenal gas. Another finding is the obliteration of the properitoneal fat stripe secondary to adjacent inflammation. CT is the imaging modality of choice to evaluate patients for the possibility of abdominal or pelvic abscess.

Bowel Obstruction   Bowel obstruction, whether partial or complete, can occur anywhere in the small or large bowel. Small-bowel diameter greater than 3 cm or large-bowel diameter greater than 5 cm is considered abnormal. Small-bowel obstructions present with air-fluid levels on upright or decubitus examinations seen in association with dilated bowel loops (Figure 4-22). In adults, the most common conditions in the differential diagnosis for obstruction include adhesions, hernias (internal or external) (Figure 4-23), and neoplasms (Table 4-4). In pediatric

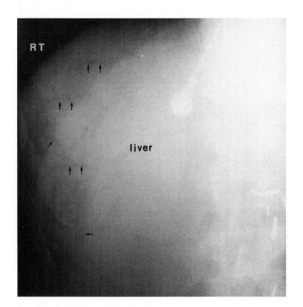

←

FIGURE 4-20 **Coned-down radiograph right upper abdomen: Portal venous air:** Irregular small branching air lucencies are seen in the periphery of the liver (arrows). This is an ominous finding, usually indicating bowel necrosis.

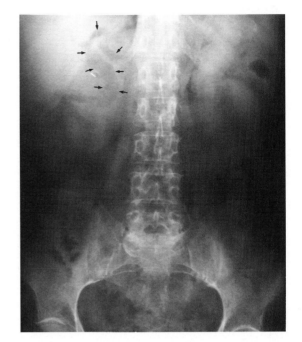

$\rightarrow$

FIGURE 4-21 Supine abdominal radiography: Biliary air: Air is present in the biliary system (arrows). Note the characteristic central location. This is a common postsurgical finding in patients who have had a prior biliary intestinal anastomosis. Biliary air also is visible in patients with a gallstone ileus or cholangitis.

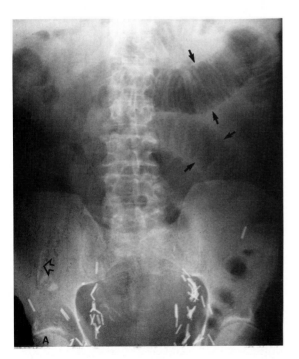

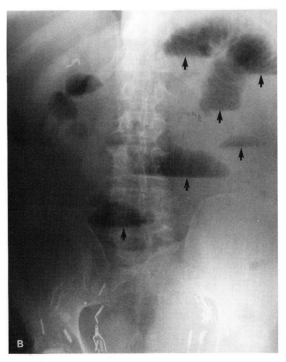

FIGURE 4-22 Supine and upright abdominal radiographs: Small-bowel obstruction: (A) Supine examination in a patient with prior bowel resection (open arrow indicates suture line) and lymph node dissection as determined by numerous pelvic surgical clips. Surgical clips are also seen in the right upper quadrant compatible with a prior cholecystectomy. Small-bowel loops are dilated (arrows) and there is a paucity of gas in the distal small bowel and colon suggesting a proximal obstruction. (B) Upright examination demonstrates numerous air fluid levels (arrows) in the dilated loops of bowel. During surgical exploration adhesions were identified as the cause of obstruction.

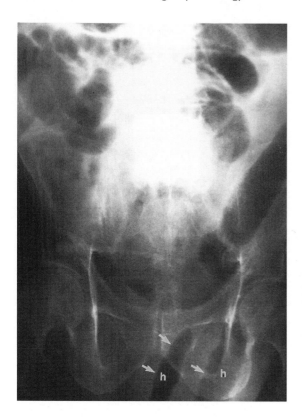

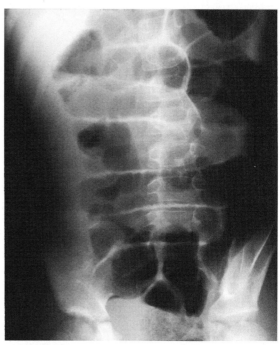

←

FIGURE 4-23   Coned-down supine lower abdominal radiograph: Inguinal hernia: Air is identified below the inguinal ligament (arrows) in small-bowel loops. This inguinal hernia (h) is large and fills the scrotum. Strangulation is a potential hazard.

→

FIGURE 4-24   Supine abdominal radiograph: Appendicitis: Numerous air-filled loops of dilated small bowel throughout the abdomen and pelvis are seen in this child. This represents a pseudo-obstruction commonly seen with acute appendicitis. Included in the differential diagnosis are intestinal intussuception and hernia.

TABLE 4-4   Differential Diagnosis of Small-Bowel Obstruction

Adhesions—prior surgery or peritonitis

Hernia

Neoplasm

Abscess

Volvulus

Intestinal foreign body or gallstone occluding lumen

Intussusception

Stricture—postinflammatory, i.e., Crohn's, postradiation

patients, intussusception, hernia, and pseudo-obstruction seen with appendicitis are the most common causes of small-bowel obstruction (Figure 4-24).

Another plain-film finding of small-bowel obstruction is a string-of-pearls sign. This is caused by small air collections in a predominantly fluid-filled obstructed bowel (Figure 4-25).

Intestinal Ileus   Intestinal ileus appears radiographically as enlargement of the GI tract. The stomach—small and large bowel—all dilate. The differential diagnosis includes trauma, medications, peritonitis, and electrolyte disturbances.

A localized ileus or sentinel loop is seen as a focal dilated loop of small bowel adjacent to an area of inflammation and can help pinpoint the potential cause. A sentinel loop can be seen in patients with cholecystitis, pancreatitis, or appendicitis (Figure 4-26).

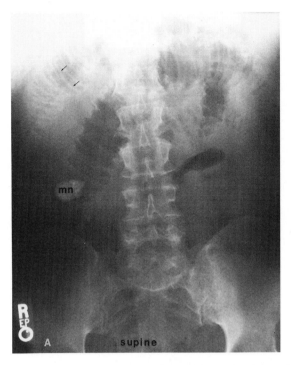 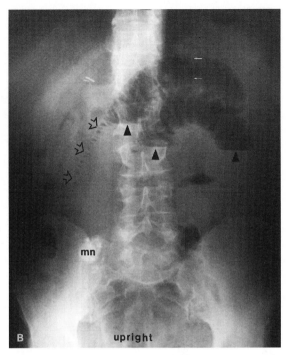

FIGURE 4-25 Supine and upright abdominal radiographs: Small-bowel obstruction, string-of-pearls sign, Calcified mesenteric lymph node: (A) Supine Examination: Numerous proximal loops of dilated small bowel are present, indicating an obstruction. Note the characteristic small-bowel valvulae conniventes (small arrows). A calcified mesenteric node (mn) is also identified. (B) Upright Examination: Numerous air-fluid levels are seen (arrowheads) in the dilated loops of small bowel. The valvulae conniventes are again identified (small arrows). Small collections of air trapped by the valvulae conniventes in the obstructed fluid-filled bowel are indicated by the open arrows. This is known as the string-of-pearls sign.

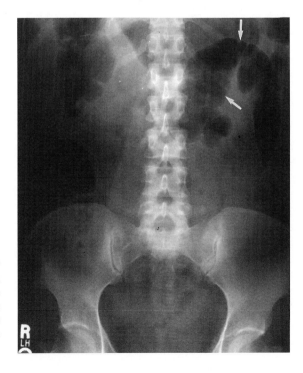

FIGURE 4-26 Supine abdominal radiograph: Sentinel loop: A focal loop of dilated small bowel is present in the left upper abdominal quadrant (arrows). This focal ileus or sentinel loop is adjacent to an inflamed pancreas in this patient with acute pancreatitis. Sentinel loops can also be seen in patients with cholecystitis and appendicitis.

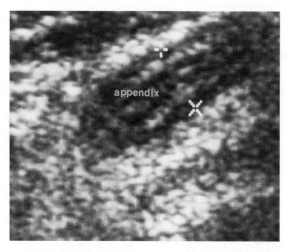

FIGURE 4-27 **Right lower quadrant ultrasound: Appendicitis:** Imaging of the right lower quadrant shows a large appendix that is not compressible. This finding, in the correct clinical setting, is highly suspicious for acute appendicitis.

Intestinal Volvulus A volvulus is a closed-loop obstruction. This means that both the afferent and efferent loops of bowel are obstructed. A volvulus can occur anywhere but is most common in the sigmoid colon and cecum. A sigmoid volvulus appears as a dilated loop of large bowel resembling an inverted U-shaped mass in the midabdominal region. A cecal volvulus occurs when the cecum twists on its mesentery. The cecum then dilates and assumes a kidney-bean shape projecting into the left upper quadrant (Figure 4-18).

Intestinal volvulus can strangulate bowel and result in ischemia and bowel necrosis. Perforation is a possible complication. Diagnosis is made by either barium enema or endoscopy.

Intussusception The vast majority of patients with intussusception are young children less than 2 years old. The cause is usually idiopathic, but this condition can be seen following upper respiratory tract infections. The child presents with crampy abdominal pain and bloody stools. Adults complain of abdominal pain and, unlike children, have a lead point, such as a polyp or tumor, causing the intussusception. Plain-film findings in both the adult and pediatric patient demonstrate a small-bowel obstruction. Children may have a lack of bowel gas in the right lower quadrant and a palpable abdominal mass on the right side. Diagnosis and treatment of pediatric intussusception is made by a single-contrast barium enema examination. Alternatively, an air-contrast examination can be performed, which, like the barium examination, is both diagnostic and potentially therapeutic.

Appendicitis Most patients with acute appendicitis have normal abdominal plain films. Occasionally, a calcified appendicolith can be identified in the right lower quadrant (Figure 4-9). This finding has a high correlation with acute appendicitis in the patient with right lower quadrant abdominal pain. Other plain-film findings suggestive of appendicitis include a localized ileus or sentinel loop in the right lower quadrant and possible obliteration of the right flank stripe. Noninvasive diagnosis of appendicitis can be made with ultrasonography as the inflamed appendix is larger than 6 mm in diameter and is not compressible (Figure 4-27).

Pancreatitis The diagnosis of pancreatitis is based on clinical and serological examinations. Imaging is usually reserved for unusual presentations of pancreatitis or cases complicated by either infection or hemorrhage.

Plain-film findings in acute pancreatitis are nonspecific. There may be a sentinel loop in the epigastric region (Figure 4-26). Amorphous calcifications are sometimes seen within the pancreas of patients with a history of chronic pancreatitis (Figure 4-11).

Acute Cholecystitis The etiology of acute cholecystitis is obstruction of the cystic duct by a gallstone. Acalculous cholecystitis is much less common and is usually seen in chronically ill patients. Plain-film findings in acute cholecystitis are nonspecific. Fewer than 15% of patients with known gallstones have calcified stones identifiable on plain film. Most gallstones are predominantly composed of cholesterol and therefore are not radiopaque. Plain films may demonstrate a localized right upper quadrant ileus.

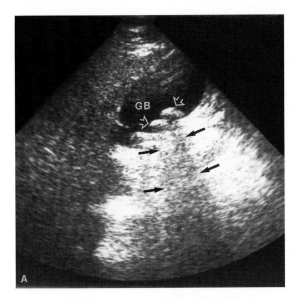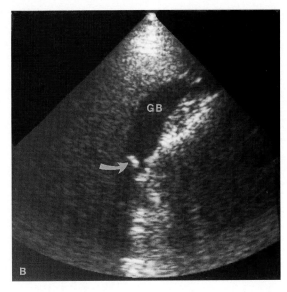

FIGURE 4-28   Ultrasound images of the gallbladder: Cholelithiasis: (A) There are two echogenic (white) gallstones (open arrows) in the gallbladder (GB) lumen. Posterior acoustical shadowing is indicated by the arrows. (B) A single gallstone (curved arrow) is lodged in the gallbladder (GB) neck.

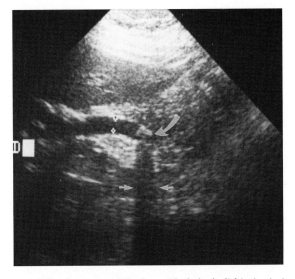

FIGURE 4-29   Ultrasound image of distal common bile duct: Choledocholithiasis: A single echogenic (white) stone is present in the dilated distal common bile duct (curved arrow). The stone demonstrates posterior acoustical shadowing (arrows).

The diagnosis of acute cholecystitis requires either ultrasonography or nuclear medicine studies. Ultrasonography is extremely sensitive in the detection of gallstones, which appear as mobile, echogenic foci in the gallbladder and demonstrate posterior acoustical shadowing (Figure 4-28). A sonographic Murphy's sign may also be present. This consists of pain localizing directly over the gallbladder. Other nonspecific sonographic findings in acute cholecystitis include fluid around the gallbladder and thickening of the gallbladder wall. Ultrasound also evaluates the intra- and extrahepatic bile ducts to exclude obstruction (Figure 4-29).

Diagnosis of acute cholecystitis with nuclear medicine is performed by intravenous injection of a radionuclide that is excreted from the liver into the biliary system and fills the gallbladder in a normal patient. However, in patients with acute cholecystitis and cystic duct obstruction, the gallbladder does not fill (Figure 4-30). Workup of the patient with RUQ pain is shown in Algorithm 4-2.

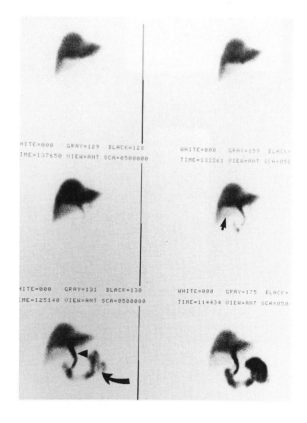

$\longrightarrow$

FIGURE 4-30 **Hepatobilliary nuclear medicine scan: Acute cholecystitis:** Multiple anterior images were obtained of the liver and biliary system. The radiotracer accumulates in the liver in a normal fashion. Delayed images show excretion of the radiotracer into the extrahepatic bile ducts (arrowhead). The gallbladder fossa shows no increase in activity (arrow). This is diagnostic of an obstructed cystic duct. Excretion of the radiotracer into the small bowel occurs in a normal fashion, demonstrating patency of the common bile duct (curved arrow).

ALGORITHM 4-2   **Evaluation of the Patient with Right Upper Quadrant Pain**

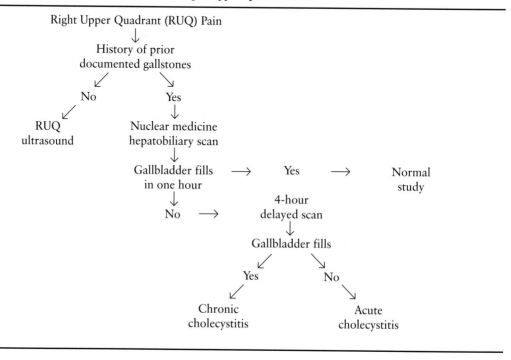

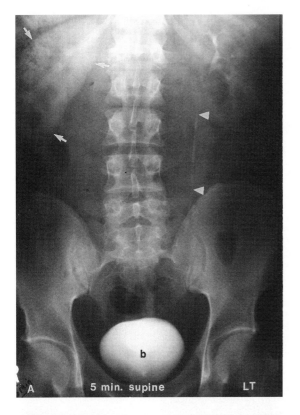

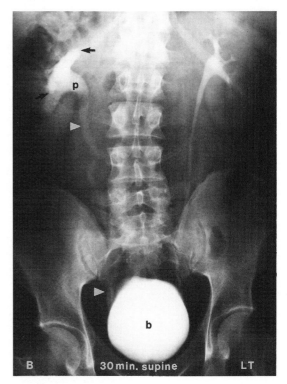

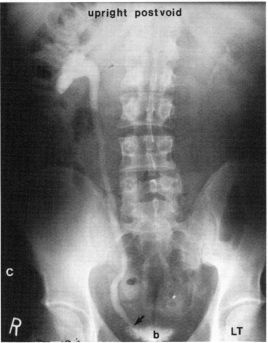

←

FIGURE 4-31   **Intravenous urogram: Distal right ureterovesical obstruction:** (A) Five-minute film obtained after the intravenous administration of iodinated contrast demonstrates a prolonged nephrogram on the right (arrows). This prolonged nephrogram indicates an obstructive process but does not identify the level of obstruction. Further delayed films are necessary. The left kidney is excreting the contrast normally down the ureter (arrowheads) into the bladder (b). (B) Thirty-minute film demonstrates a dilated right renal pelvis (p). The calyces are blunted (arrows) indicating hydronephrosis. The right ureter is dilated (arrowheads) and opacified to the level of the bladder (b). The left calyces, pelvis, and ureter are normal. (C) Upright postvoid examination demonstrates persistent dilatation of the contrast-filled, right ureter. This is known as a standing column of contrast. After the bladder (b) is emptied, the level of obstruction is easily identified as the ureterovesical junction (arrow). The left side is barely visible as it emptied normally.

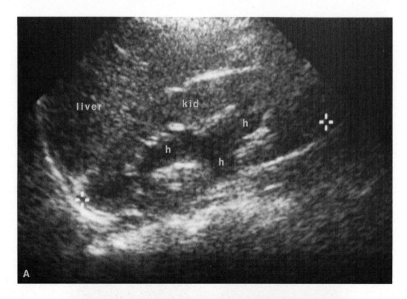

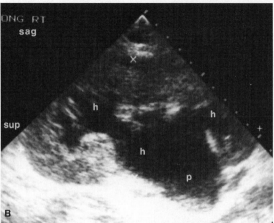

FIGURE 4-32 Sagittal renal ultrasound images: Hydronephrosis (two cases): (A) The right kidney (kid) is identified in close approximation to the liver. The central renal sinus is sonolucent (dark) and dilated, diagnostic of mild hydronephrosis (h). (B) Moderate hydronephrosis (h) is present with dilatation of the renal pelvis (p).

GENITOURINARY TRACT

Nephrolithiasis

Renal calculi commonly contain calcium, and the majority (approximately 85%) are identifiable on plain films of the abdomen. Other stones composed of uric acid are not visible on plain films. Patients presenting with flank pain and hematuria are frequently evaluated with an intravenous urogram (IVU) to exclude an obstructing ureteral stone. Occasionally patients with complete ureteral obstruction will present with flank pain without hematuria. Renal stones usually obstruct at one of three areas: the ureteropelvic junction, the pelvic brim, or the ureterovesical junction.

The IVU is obtained to identify the level of obstruction. Diagnostic keys to identifying obstruction on IVU include a delayed nephrogram, dilatation of the renal collecting systems (hydronephrosis), and the presence of a column of contrast in the obstructed ureter on postvoid upright examination (Figure 4-31).

Patients who are allergic to iodinated contrast can be evaluated with ultrasonography to exclude hydronephrosis (Figure 4-32) or any renal stones (Figure 4-33). Plain films of the abdomen can be used to detect any potentially obstructing calcified stones.

Stag-horn calculi are very characteristic stones seen in patients with chronic urinary tract infections. They commonly fill renal calyces or even the renal pelvis (Figure 4-34).

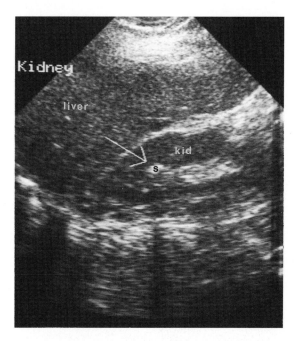

FIGURE 4-33 Sagittal renal ultrasound: Renal stone: A small echogenic (white) stone (s) is identified in the superior pole of the right kidney (kid) by the arrow. Note the posterior acoustical shadowing.

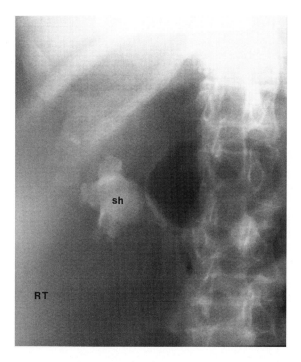

FIGURE 4-34 Coned-down radiograph right renal fossa: Staghorn calculus: A staghorn (sh) calculus is identified in the right renal pelvis. These stones characteristically mold themselves into the shape of the renal collecting system and are the sequelae of chronic infection.

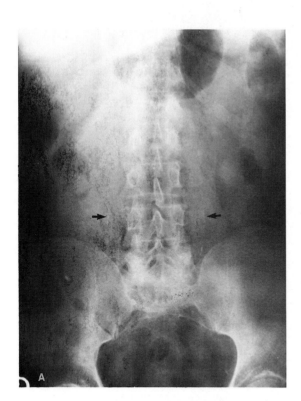 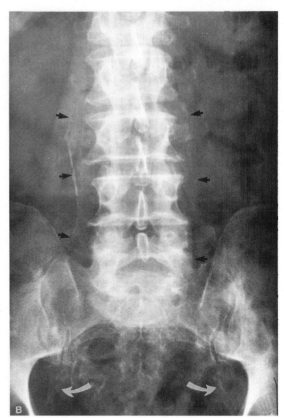

FIGURE 4-35   **Supine abdominal radiograph: Abdominal aortic aneurysm (2 cases):** (A) Linear calcifications are identified lateral to each side of the lumbar spine (arrows). These calcifications represent atherosclerotic disease of the abdominal aorta. There is an aneurysm present as the distance between the calcifications exceeds 3 cm. (B) Different patient illustrating another abdominal aortic aneurysm. Calcific atherosclerotic disease is present (arrows) outlining the aortic aneurysm. This disease extends into the common iliac arteries (curved arrows).

Hydronephrosis

Hydronephrosis is defined as distention of the renal pelvis and calices secondary to urinary tract obstruction. This obstruction may be due to either stone disease, strictures, or tumors. Hydronephrosis is demonstrated on ultrasound as areas of dark or anechoic urine filling a dilated collecting system (Figure 4-32).

Abdominal Aortic Aneurysm

Aneurysm of the abdominal aorta is defined as a transverse measurement greater than 3 cm. Abdominal aortic aneurysms are associated with atherosclerotic calcifications that are easily identifiable on plain film (Figure 4-35). Other imaging modalities, including ultrasonography and CT, are sensitive in measuring the diameter of the abdominal aorta. CT is, however, more sensitive in detecting any associated hemorrhage (Figure 4-36).

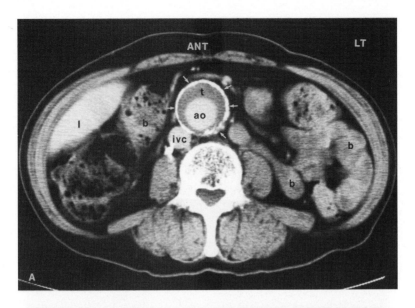

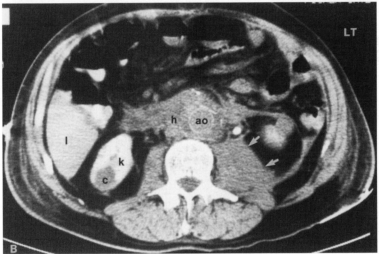

FIGURE 4-36   **Abdominal CT: Abdominal aortic aneurysm and leaking aneurysm:** (A) Axial image of the abdomen obtained below the level of the kidneys. There is contrast enhancement of the liver (l), inferior vena cava (ivc), and aorta (ao). Nonopacified bowel (b) is seen throughout the abdomen. Circumferential high attenuation calcium is seen in the wall of the abdominal aorta (arrows). The diameter of the aorta exceeds 3 cm, diagnostic of an aneurysm. There is associated thrombus (t) in the aortic lumen. (B) Different patient than A. The aorta (ao) is surrounded by low-attenuation hemorrhage (h) from a leaking aneurysm. The hemorrhage extends into the left perirenal space (arrows). The liver (l) and right kidney (k) demonstrate normal enhancement. There is a simple cyst (c) present on the kidney.

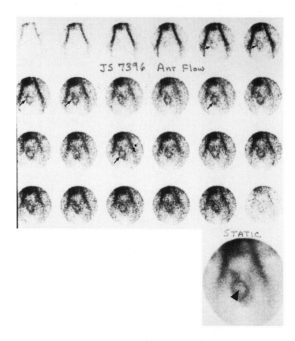

FIGURE 4-37 Radionuclide imaging testes: Missed testicular torsion: Radionuclide perfusion examination of the testes demonstrates increased perfusion to the right hemiscrotum (arrows). Static image shows a ring of increased activity representing reactive hyperemia around a central cold defect that corresponds to an infarcted testicle (arrowhead) that resulted from torsion. Testicular scans are ordered to differentiate epididymitis from a missed testicular torsion.

GENITOURINARY NONTRAUMATIC EMERGENCIES

Testicular Torsion

Young men presenting with acute testicular pain are evaluated for the possibility of testicular torsion. The differential diagnosis includes acute epididymitis. The distinction between the two is clinically difficult to make. Diagnosis can be made with either ultrasonography or radionuclide flow studies (Figure 4-37).

Ovarian Torsion

Ovarian torsion occurs when an ovary, usually diseased, rotates on its vascular axis. This results in a compromised vascular supply and ischemia. The diagnosis can be difficult to make, but ultrasonography does demonstrate an enlarged hypoechoic edematous ovary. Doppler interrogation of the adjacent vascular structures demonstrates absent flow.

Pelvic Inflammatory Disease

The sexually transmitted diseases gonorrhea and chlamydia are two organisms responsible for causing pelvic inflammatory disease (PID). Ultrasonography is the imaging modality of choice in the evaluation of a patient with pelvic pain, fever, and leukocytosis. Ultrasonographic findings of PID represent a spectrum from normal to grossly abnormal. Fluid in the cul-de-sac as well as dilatation of the fallopian tubes and adnexal masses are possible findings.

Ectopic Pregnancy

Women presenting with vaginal bleeding, pelvic pain, or hypotension should have an emergent pregnancy test performed. If the test is positive, then an ectopic pregnancy needs to be excluded. Patients who are at risk for ectopic pregnancy include women who have had a history of prior pelvic inflammatory disease, previous tubal ligation, women utilizing intrauterine devices for contraception, and women who are taking fertility drugs.

The diagnosis of ectopic pregnancy is based on the pregnancy test, ultrasonographic findings, and physical examination. An approach to evaluating the patient with a suspected ectopic pregnancy is described in Algorithm 4-3.

ALGORITHM 4-3   Evaluation of the Patient with a Suspected Ectopic Pregnancy

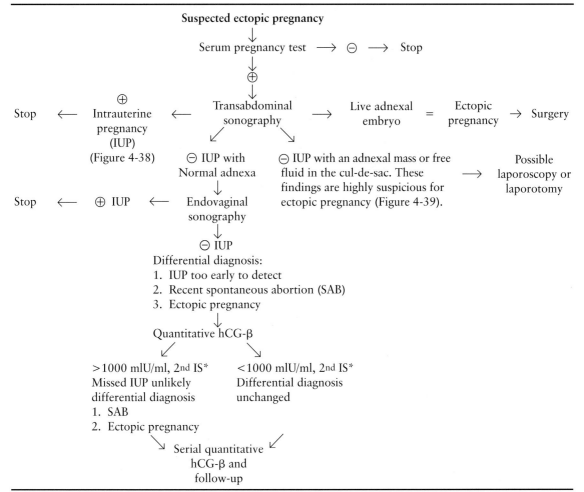

Suspected ectopic pregnancy

Serum pregnancy test ⟶ ⊖ ⟶ Stop

⊕

Transabdominal sonography ⟶ Live adnexal embryo = Ectopic pregnancy → Surgery

Stop ← Intrauterine pregnancy (IUP) (Figure 4-38) ← ⊕

⊖ IUP with Normal adnexa

⊖ IUP with an adnexal mass or free fluid in the cul-de-sac. These findings are highly suspicious for ectopic pregnancy (Figure 4-39). ⟶ Possible laparoscopy or laparotomy

Stop ← ⊕ IUP ← Endovaginal sonography

⊖ IUP

Differential diagnosis:
1. IUP too early to detect
2. Recent spontaneous abortion (SAB)
3. Ectopic pregnancy

Quantitative hCG-β

>1000 mlU/ml, 2nd IS*
Missed IUP unlikely
differential diagnosis
1. SAB
2. Ectopic pregnancy

<1000 mlU/ml, 2nd IS*
Differential diagnosis
unchanged

Serial quantitative hCG-β and follow-up

*2nd IS = Second International standard.

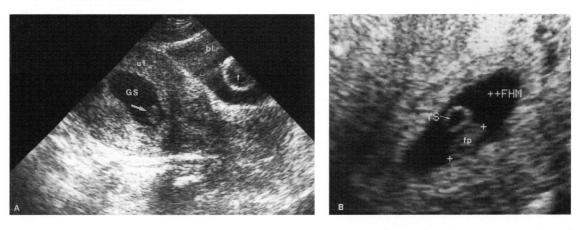

FIGURE 4-38   Pelvic ultrasound: Normal intrauterine pregnancy: (A) A sagittal image through the uterus was obtained in this young female to exclude an ectopic pregnancy. A gestational sac (GS) is identified in the uterus (ut). Within the sac is a fetal pole (arrow). The bladder (bl) was filled by instilling fluid through the patient's Foley catheter (f). (B) Further information was obtained repeating the examination with an endovaginal transducer. Close-up of the gestational sac shows a live fetal pole (fp) and fetal heart motion (FHM). The normal yolk sac (YS) is seen adjacent to the fetal pole. These findings are diagnostic of a live intrauterine pregnancy. The possibility of a coexistent ectopic gestation is approximately 1 in 30,000.

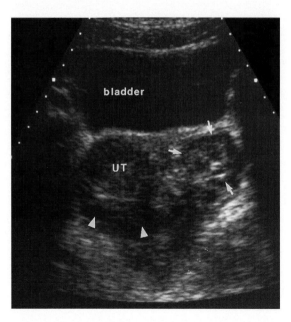

FIGURE 4-39 **Transabdominal pelvic ultrasound: Ectopic pregnancy:** Transverse pelvic ultrasound of this young female with pelvic pain and a positive pregnancy test demonstrates a complex adnexal mass (arrows) adjacent to her uterus (UT). Fluid is visible in the cul-de-sac (arrowheads). These findings are strongly indicative of an ectopic pregnancy and in this case was confirmed by laparoscopy.

Chapter 4 Abdominal Pearls _____

1. Pneumoperitoneum may be difficult to diagnose on supine examinations.
2. Don't confuse colonic interposition with pneumoperitoneum.
3. Portal venous gas is an ominous sign that can be difficult to detect without adequate films and careful observation.
4. Complete ureteral obstruction from a stone occasionally presents without hematuria.
5. Do not delay the diagnostic evaluation of a patient with a suspected testicular torsion.
6. A positive pregnancy test without a documented intrauterine pregnancy is an ectopic pregnancy until proven otherwise.
7. Female patients with PID may present with RUQ pain secondary to perihepatitis.
8. Children with lower lobe pneumonias can present to the emergency department with abdominal pain.
9. Bilious vomiting in a newborn is an ominous sign. Exclude midgut volvulus and sepsis.
10. Do not catheterize a trauma patient who has blood at the urethral meatus without first clearing the urethra with a retrograde urethrogram.
11. Feculent emesis suggests a bowel obstruction.

Chapter

5

Orthopedic Radiology

OVERVIEW

Emergency physicians request countless skeletal radiographs each year to "rule out fracture" in trauma patients. Perhaps they are aware that the number-one reason for lawsuits in their profession is a missed fracture.

When ordering radiographs of the extremities, it is important to obtain a minimum of two perpendicular views, usually an anteroposterior and a lateral projection. Additional oblique views should be obtained when radiographing the wrist, hand, ankle, and foot. Limiting the radiographic examination to a single view may lead to misdiagnosis or failure to adequately characterize a known fracture (Figure 5-1). Unless there is a possibility of neurovascular injury, an attempt to take two views should be made. Films should be of high quality and the patient should be positioned appropriately.

TECHNIQUES
Plain Film

Plain films are the mainstay in both detecting and characterizing the vast majority of fractures and dislocations.

Computed Tomography (CT)   Computed tomography's greatest use outside of neuroradiology applications is in the evaluation of pelvic fractures. CT evaluation of complicated joint fractures may also be of benefit preoperatively.

Magnetic Resonance Imaging (MRI)   MRI has limited usefulness in the evaluation of acute extremity trauma with the exception of detecting occult hip fractures. It does, however, provide useful information when evaluating joint trauma, suspected bone tumors, osteomyelitis, or avascular necrosis.

Conventional Tomography   Conventional tomography is performed using complex movements of the X-ray tube and X-ray film cassette. Images can be obtained in small incremental measurements in multiple planes of imaging. This can be a useful technique when evaluating fractures involving joints and the spine. This technique has largely been replaced by thin section CT with multiplanar image reconstruction.

EVALUATION OF ABNORMAL PLAIN FILMS

Many pathologic entities that affect the musculoskeletal system are subtle. When a diagnosis is not readily apparent, additional imaging techniques and consultation with orthopedic specialists may be necessary. The emergency physician who sees a bone abnormality on plain film, should answer the following three questions.

First, does the finding indicate an acute fracture? The spectrum of fractures ranges from undetectable to grossly deformed. For this reason, attention should be paid to particular clues when examining the films. Most fractures in adults traverse the cortical surfaces, leading to a complete cortical break. However, with impaction injuries, there may be nothing more than an increased area of bone density, representing fractured and compressed bony trabeculae. Fracture margins are sharp or ill-defined but not well corticated. This helps distinguish an acute injury from an old, healed fracture (Figure 5-2) or normal accessory ossification center (Figure 5-3). Soft-tissue signs indicative of a fracture include swelling and obliteration of fascial planes. These signs are absent in insignificant or old trauma. Additional soft-tissue indicators of an acute fracture are seen with joint trauma. These include a fat/blood

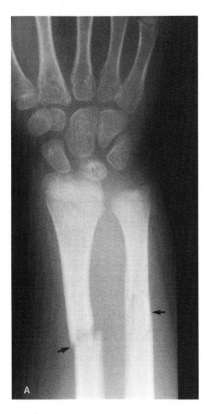

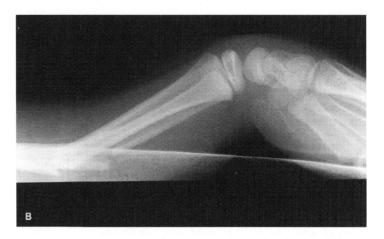

FIGURE 5-1 **AP and lateral wrist: Angulated forearm fracture:** (A) The AP view shows a distal forearm fracture (arrows). (B) The lateral projection demonstrates marked anterior apex angulation at the fracture site. The AP view does not reveal the fracture angulation. Although in this case the deformity is clinically apparent, in other instances subtle angular deformities can be missed without two perpendicular views.

FIGURE 5-2 **Detail view distal ulna (2) cases: Acute versus old trauma:** In (A), there is an acute ulnar styloid fracture (arrows). The fracture margins are indistinct, and the soft tissues are swollen (dashed line). (B) A different patient shows evidence of an old ulnar styloid fracture. The fracture margins are well corticated and the soft tissues are normal.

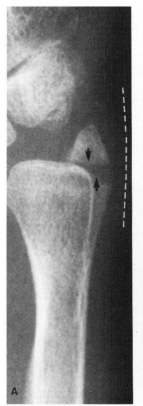
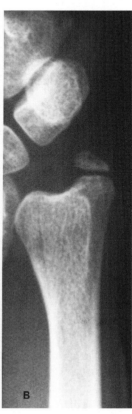

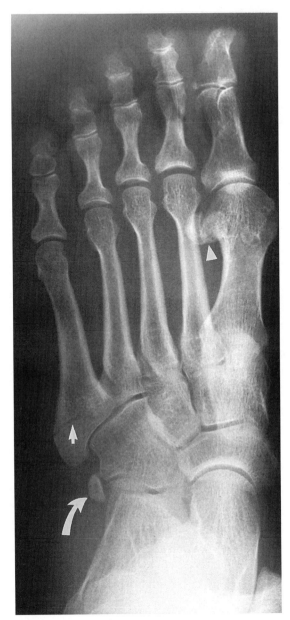

FIGURE 5-3   **Oblique view foot: Acute fracture and fracture simulators:** There is a nondisplaced transverse fracture of the proximal fifth metatarsal (arrow). A secondary ossification center (curved arrow) and normal sesamoid bones (arrowhead) are present and should not be confused with acute fracture fragments.

TABLE 5-1   Easily Missed Fractures and Techniques to Avoid Misdiagnosis

Easily Missed Fractures	Diagnostic Key/Further Work-up
Clavicle	Apical lordotic radiographs for difficult cases.
Sternoclavicular joint	Thin-section CT through the sternoclavicular joint with coronal reconstruction.
Elbow	Careful attention to anterior humeral line, radiocapitellar line and fat pads.
Scaphoid	Additional scaphoid views or bone scan.
Carpal bone dislocations	Careful attention to alignment of radius, capitate, and lunate on lateral wrist plain films.
Femoral neck	Radionuclide bone scan or MRI.
Sacrum	Sacral ala intact, SI joints symmetric. Additional imaging with CT or bone scan.
Osteochondral injuries	CT or MRI.
Distal fibula	Careful attention to appearance on lateral films.
Posterior tibial lip	Careful attention to appearance on lateral films.
Lisfranc foot injury	Assure normal alignment of the first and second metatarsal bones with the medial and middle cuneiform bones.

level (lipohemarthrosis) and displaced fat pads. Easily missed fractures and techniques to assist in making a correct diagnosis are included in Table 5-1.

Acute fractures can sometimes be difficult to detect in osteoporotic patients or patients with severe degenerative disease. In these circumstances, and others where the clinical suspicion for fracture is high and the plain films are normal, the emergency physician should remain suspicious and refer the patient for appropriate follow-up. If old films of the traumatized area are available, they may be helpful in deciphering the radiographs in question.

Using a fracture eponym (i.e., Colles' fracture) is only useful when everyone involved in the care of the patient understands the terminology. There are numerous fracture eponyms. Some are obscure names that may lead to their inappropriate usage and clinical confusion. Some common eponyms are

listed throughout this chapter for purposes of completeness. However, it is more appropriate to describe a fracture as listed in Table 5-2.

Pediatric patients present additional difficulties in radiographic interpretation of bone abnormalities. Numerous growth centers throughout the body can cause diagnostic confusion. The appearance of normal juvenile physeal centers varies according to the patient's age and sex. Reference to a textbook of normal radiographic anatomy/variants is very useful. If clinical confusion persists, then contralateral films for comparison may help.

Sesamoid bones and accessory (secondary) ossification centers have characteristic locations and appearances. Both are most numerous in the hands and feet. Again, referencing a textbook of normal variants is essential. Evaluation of a patient with a suspected fracture is included in Algorithm 5-1.

TABLE 5-2   Fracture Description

1. Complete or incomplete cortical break
2. Fracture plane
   a. Transverse
   b. Oblique
   c. Spiral
   d. Avulsion
   e. Mixed transverse—oblique
3. Displacement of the distal fragment in relation to the proximal fragment, anterior, medial, radial, etc.
4. Angulation—Described according to the direction of the fracture angle apex, i.e., dorsal apex angulation
5. Limb shortening or overriding of bony fragments
6. Comminution
7. Other considerations
   a. Intra-articular extension
   b. Associated subluxations/dislocations
   c. Soft-tissue foreign bodies
   d. Involvement of physis (pediatric fractures)

ALGORITHM 5-1   Work-up of a Suspected Fracture

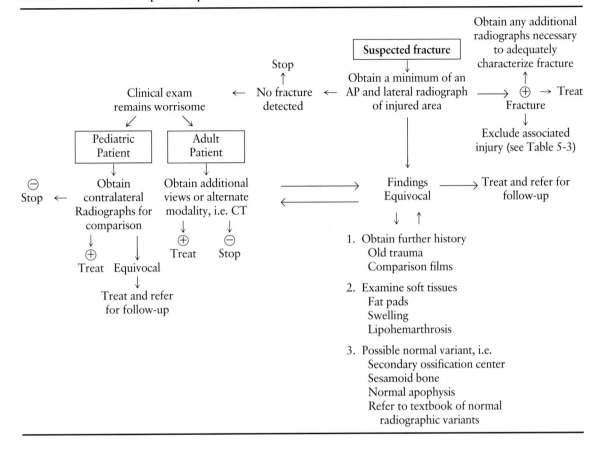

TABLE 5-3   Common Fractures and Their Associated Injuries

Fracture	Associated Injuries
Clavicle	Scapula, chest, i.e., hemothorax or pneumothorax
Upper rib	Vascular trauma, i.e., aorta, great vessels
Lower rib	Intra-abdominal trauma, i.e., splenic, hepatic, or renal injury
Pelvis	Genitourinary and neurovascular injury
Femur	Hip dislocation
Calcaneus	Spinal injury, especially lumbar spine. Contralateral foot and ankle injuries.

The second question that needs to be answered is: is the finding suspicious for a bone tumor? If this question cannot be answered in the negative, then the patient needs an appropriate referral. Plain-film findings that are suspicious include:

1. Areas of bone sclerosis or lysis.
2. Periosteal changes.
3. Expansile lesions or evidence of cortical disruption.
4. An associated soft-tissue mass.

In general, bone tumors are rare. Metastatic disease is more common in patients more than 40 years old. An adult with a lytic bone lesion is worrisome for a metastatic deposit from lung, kidney, breast, or thyroid cancer (Figure 5-4). If the lesion is sclerotic, then metastatic prostate cancer is the most common cause in men and metastatic breast cancer is the most common cause in women (Figure 5-5).

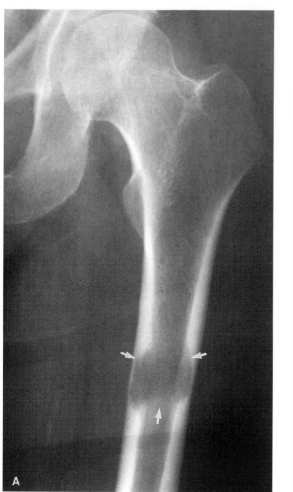

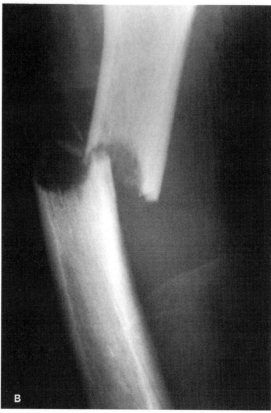

FIGURE 5-4 **Detail view of the proximal femur: Pathologic fracture:** (A) AP view of the hip shows a lytic bone lesion in the proximal femoral shaft (arrows). The margins of this lesion are poorly defined and there is evidence of cortical thinning. This lesion represents metastasis from the patient's lung carcinoma. Before proper therapy could be instituted, the patient returned to the emergency department with acute hip pain. (B) Repeat radiographs demonstrate a pathologic fracture has occurred through the lesion.

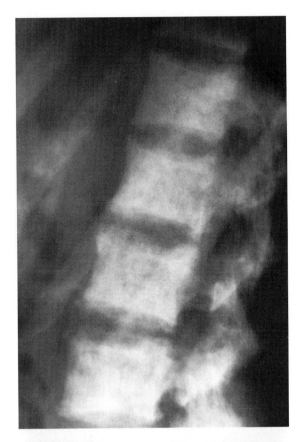

FIGURE 5-5   Detail lateral view thoracolumbar spine: Metastatic prostate cancer: The vertebral bodies are all diffusely sclerotic, representing metastatic prostate cancer. If this was a female patient, metastatic breast cancer would be the most likely diagnosis.

→

FIGURE 5-6   AP and lateral knee: Osteosarcoma: AP (A) and lateral (B) projections of the knee show a mixed lytic and sclerotic lesion of the distal femur in this child. This is the typical location and appearance for an osteosarcoma.

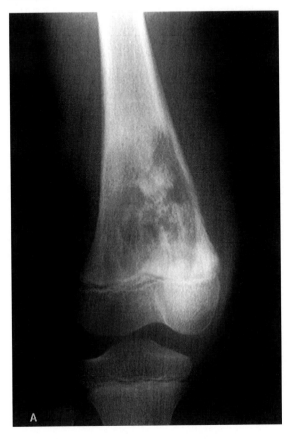

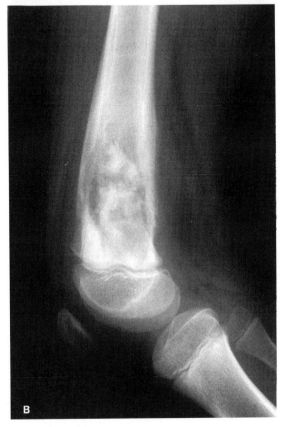

Primary osteosarcomas occur most commonly in patients less than 25 years old. They are frequently located in the distal femur, proximal tibia, or proximal humerus. Of the four histologic types, the mixed osteolytic/blastic form is the most common (Figure 5-6).

There are a few well-known benign bone lesions that require no additional tests or follow-up. It is important to be able to recognize bone islands, fibrous cortical defects, and nonossifying fibromas as common lesions found incidentally on extremity radiographs. Bone islands appear as a cortically based sclerotic focus less than 1.5 cm in size. They are usually round or elliptical in shape, are aligned with the trabeculae, and have an irregular margin with small spicules extending into adjacent bone (Figure 5-7). Fibrous cortical defects and nonossifying fibromas are pathologically the same except for size. Both are lucent lesions with a sclerotic rim located most commonly in the metaphysis of the distal femur, tibia, and fibula. Lesions less than 1.5 cm in size are

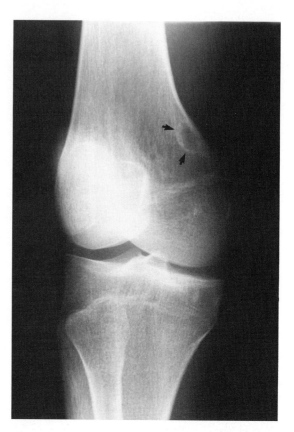

FIGURE 5-8   Oblique view knee: Fibrous cortical defect: There is a small lucent lesion of the distal femoral cortex (arrows). The borders are sclerotic. This is the characteristic location and appearance of a fibrous cortical defect. These lesions are pathologically the same as nonossifying fibromas except for size. It is important to remember that these lesions are asymptomatic with no associated periosteal reaction. These lesions eventually disappear and are not seen in patients older than 30 years of age.

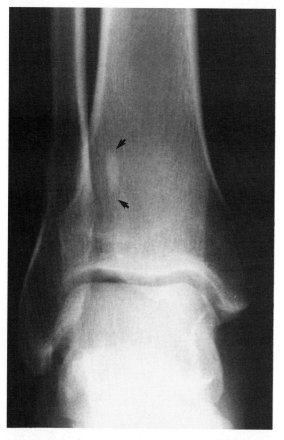

FIGURE 5-7   AP ankle: Benign bone island: There is a small sclerotic lesion in the distal tibial metaphysis (arrows). This has all the characteristics of a benign bone island. It is aligned with the trabeculae and has an irregular margin with small spicules.

called fibrous cortical defects (Figure 5-8). A larger lesion is a nonossifying fibroma (NOF). These lesions are common in children and adolescents but are rare in adults. It is important to note that these lesions are asymptomatic, and no periosteal changes are present. Pathologic fractures can occur through large NOFs (Figure 5-9).

The third question to answer is, could the finding represent osteomyelitis?

Some patients with osteomyelitis will have a history of bone pain, fever, leukocytosis, and plain films showing a destructive bone lesion. Unfortunately, plain films are usually not helpful early in the course of the disease and may not show any abnormality for up to 2 weeks after the onset of infection. The first radiographic manifestation is usually soft-tissue swelling, followed by bone destruction and periosteal reaction (Figure 5-10). The periosteal

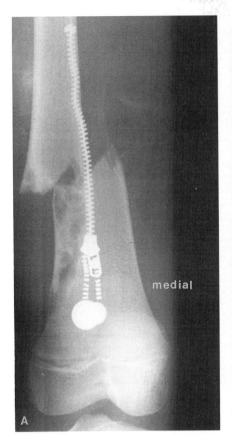

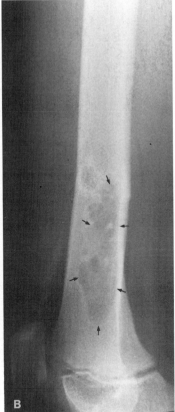

←

FIGURE 5-9 **AP and lateral distal femur: Pathologic fracture through a nonossifying fibrous (NOF):** (A) AP view shows a transverse fracture through a large lucent lesion (NOF) in the distal femoral diametaphyseal region. The distal fragment is displaced medially. The NOF is partially obscured on the AP view by a zipper on the air splint, but is well seen on the lateral view (B) (arrows).

FIGURE 5-10 **Detail view toes: Osteomyelitis:** (A) Detail view toes shows possible narrowing of the interphalangeal joint of the great toe. Soft tissues are swollen (arrows). (B) Same patient 10 days later demonstrates marked bony destruction of the great toe. It is important to diagnose osteomyelitis early and not wait for the late radiographic findings of bone destruction. If the clinical and laboratory data is equivocal, then a nuclear medicine bone scan or MRI is warranted.

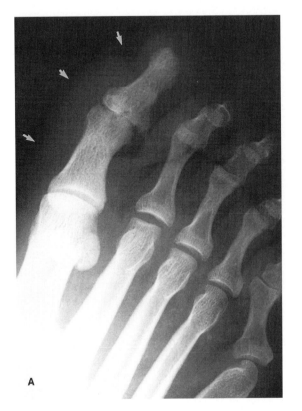

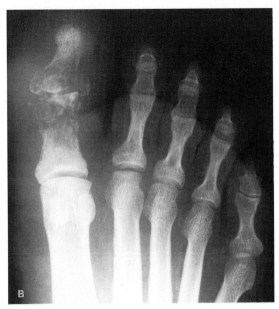

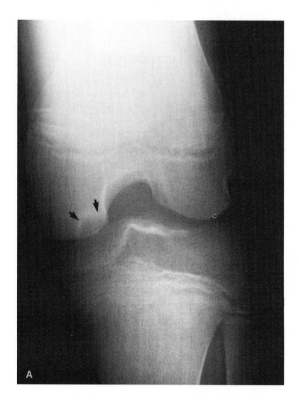
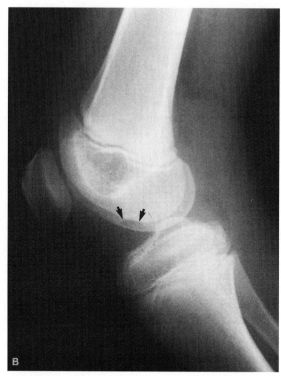

FIGURE 5-11   Tunnel and lateral views of the knee: Osteochondral fracture: (A) Tunnel view shows a crescent-shaped defect of the medial epicondyle (arrows). (B) The lateral view demonstrates the osteochondral fracture as a depression in the condyle (arrows). These fractures are easily overlooked and careful inspection of the articular surfaces is required to avoid misdiagnosis.

reaction may precede the bone destruction if the osteomyelitis is secondary to an adjacent infection. *Staphylococcal aureus* is a common organism causing osteomyelitis and may infect the bone by direct inoculation or hematogenous spread. Extension of an adjacent cellulitis to bone is another route of infection commonly seen in diabetics with foot ulcers. Early osteomyelitis can be diagnosed with MRI or nuclear medicine studies.

SPECIAL ORTHOPEDIC CONSIDERATIONS

Osteochondral Fractures

Trauma to a joint may result in injury to cartilage and underlying bone. In the knee, this can be seen following patellar dislocation. Radiographically, these osteochondral fractures are difficult to detect but appear as a crescent-shaped defect at the site of trauma (Figures 5-11, 5-12). Intra-articular cartilage fragments can move around the affected joint and cause problems with movement (i.e., "locking"). Furthermore, they can eventually calcify and be seen on plain films.

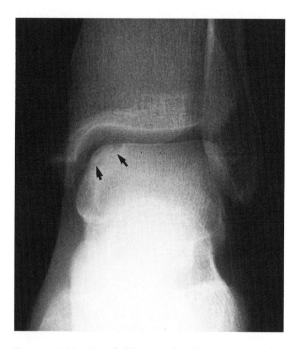

FIGURE 5-12   Detail AP view of ankle: Osteochondral fracture of the talar dome: Osteochondral fracture of the medial talar dome (arrow) is seen in this patient after a twisting injury.

Stress Fractures

Patients classically have pain in the region of the second and third metatarsals following strenuous repetitive activity. Radiographically, the bones may appear normal during the acute phase. After 2 to 3 weeks, plain films demonstrate callus forming around the stress fracture (Figure 5-13). Other common sites for stress fractures include the calcaneus (Figure 5-14) as well as the proximal and distal aspects of the tibia and fibula. If the diagnosis is suspected but not confirmed on plain films, a radionuclide bone scan will demonstrate an area of increased radiotracer labeling in the involved bone.

Pathologic Fractures

Pathologic fractures occur through areas of abnormal bone. In adults, pathologic fractures usually occur in bone involved with metastatic tumor (Figure 5-4). Clinically, a pathologic fracture should be suspected when the patient reports a history of pain

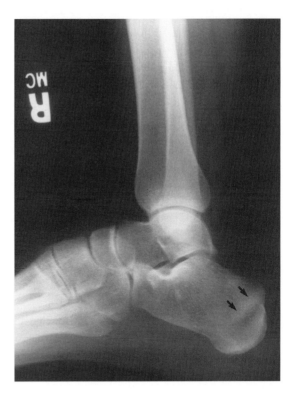

FIGURE 5-14 Lateral view ankle: Stress fracture calcaneus: Arrows indicate a linear area of sclerosis in the posterior calcaneus. Radionuclide bone scan showed abnormal uptake in this area confirming a healing stress fracture.

or swelling in the area prior to the injury and a relatively insignificant amount of trauma resulted in the fracture. Radiographically, pathologic fractures are characterized by a fracture across an area of abnormal bone. The abnormality may consist of cortical thinning, cortical expansion, or cortical destruction. Transverse fractures outside of the bony diaphysis should raise suspicion. Compression fractures of the adult spine in the absence of trauma are frequently seen in patients with multiple myeloma and osteoporosis. Childhood pathologic fractures are uncommon and are usually due to underlying benign bony abnormalities such as nonossifying fibromas (Figure 5-9) or simple bone cysts. Pediatric vertebral body compression fractures should suggest the possibility of child abuse or a systemic abnormality such as leukemia or eosinophilic granuloma.

ORTHOPEDIC CONSIDERATIONS IN THE PEDIATRIC POPULATION

Children are cartilaginous structures that ossify with increasing age. Therefore, they commonly present with incomplete fractures that are classified according to their appearance (Figure 5-15). Greenstick fractures result in a complete fracture of one

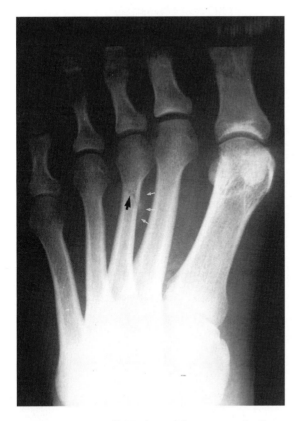

FIGURE 5-13 Detail AP view of the metatarsals: Stress fracture: This jogger continued to run on a painful foot. AP radiograph shows a stress fracture of the distal third metatarsal (arrow). Callus is present around the fracture indicating healing and is evidence that this is a subacute injury (small arrows).

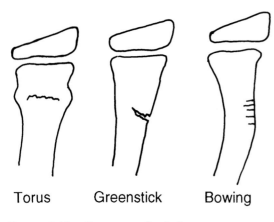

Torus   Greenstick   Bowing

FIGURE 5-15   Common pediatric fractures.

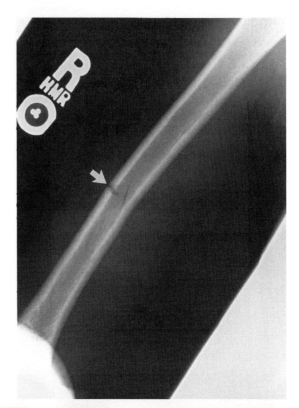

→

FIGURE 5-16   **AP humerus: Green-stick fracture:** AP humerus radiograph shows an incomplete transverse midshaft fracture (arrow). This is a classic green-stick fracture, so named because the break is similar to that of a green twig. This type of fracture commonly involves the radius, ulna, and clavicle.

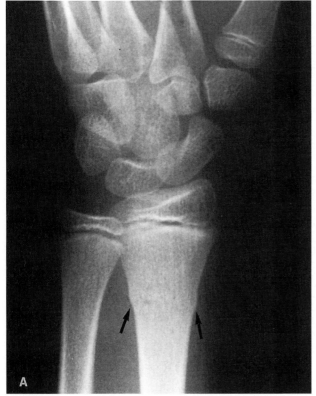

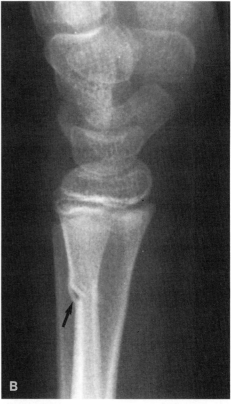

FIGURE 5-17   **AP and lateral wrist: Torus fracture of the radius:** Torus fractures commonly involve the metaphysis of long bones such as the radius and ulna. (A) The AP view shows subtle buckling of the medial and lateral cortex of the distal radius (arrows). (B) Dorsal buckling is evident on the lateral projection (arrow).

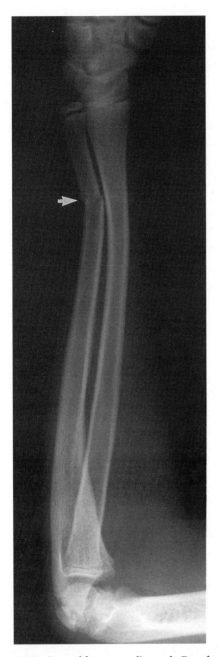

FIGURE 5-18 **Lateral forearm radiograph: Bow fracture of the radius:** There is a distal ulna fracture (arrow) associated with a bow fracture of the radius. The bow injury usually affects the entire length of bone and is a common injury of the radius, ulna, and fibula. If there is any clinical doubt about the diagnosis, contralateral radiographs would be helpful.

Type		Incidence
I		6%
II		75%
III		8%
IV		10%
V		1%

e=epiphysis
m=metaphysis

FIGURE 5-19 Salter-Harris classification of epiphyseal injuries.

the torus fracture of the distal forearm (Figure 5-17). Bow fractures are easily overlooked as the cortex is grossly intact and no definite buckling can be seen (Figure 5-18). When clinical suspicion is high, contralateral radiographs will demonstrate the abnormal bending of the affected bone.

Fractures Involving Growth Centers

Fractures of the epiphyseal complex can involve the metaphysis, physis, and not uncommonly the epiphysis. Salter-Harris classification is used to characterize these injuries and assist in determining both appropriate therapy and possible complications (Figure 5-19). Type II Salter-Harris injuries are the most common (Figure 5-20), and Type V injuries are the least common. Salter-Harris Type I or V can be difficult to detect on initial radiographs. Follow-up films may demonstrate healing bone (Figure 5-21). While the epiphysis adds to bone length, the apophysis serves as a site of muscular attachment. Apophyseal injuries are the result of avulsive forces occurring with strenuous muscular activity. The injured apophysis becomes displaced from its

cortical margin with bending and compression of the other bony cortex (Figure 5-16). Torus fractures are the result of compressive forces and are manifested radiographically by cortical buckling in the metaphyseal region of the long bone. The most common fracture of the upper extremity in childhood is

FIGURE 5-20 **Detail view 5th finger: Salter-Harris II fracture proximal phalanx:** A Salter-Harris II fracture is present at the base of the fifth proximal phalanx. A fragment of the metaphysis (m) is seen with the displaced epiphysis (e) (arrow). This is referred to as a corner sign and helps make the diagnosis. Salter-Harris II fractures are the most common epiphyseal injury and frequently involve the distal long bones such as the radius, ulna, femur, and tibia.

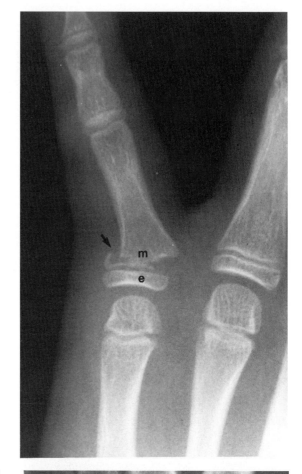

FIGURE 5-21 **AP wrist films, initial and follow-up: Healing distal radial fracture:** (A) Initial film is normal in this adolescent with wrist trauma. (B) Two-week follow-up exam shows an area of sclerosis involving the physis. This probably represents a healing Salter-Harris type V injury. This example illustrates the importance of follow-up examinations in diagnosing occult skeletal trauma.

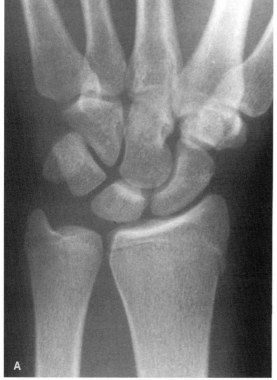

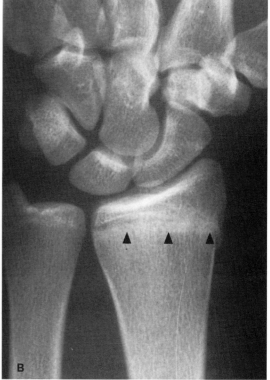

FIGURE 5-22 **Detail view juvenile pelvis: Normal apophysis:** The normal ischial tuberosity apophysis is seen bilaterally in this child (arrows). Avulsion forces can displace the normal apophysis, and direct comparison to the contralateral side is important in making the diagnosis. Apophyseal injuries are common in adolescent athletes. Other pelvic apophyseal centers that are frequently injured are the anterior superior/inferior iliac spines.

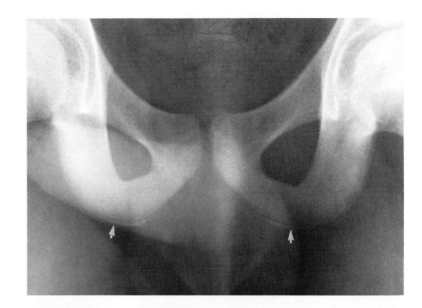

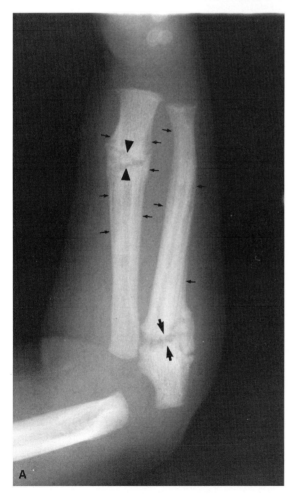

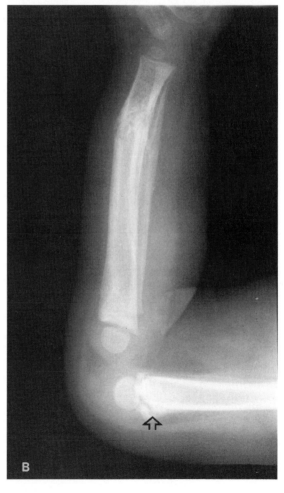

FIGURE 5-23 **AP, lateral forearm: Numerous fractures; child abuse:** (A) The AP forearm shows the characteristic findings diagnostic of child abuse. There are numerous fractures in various stages of healing. The proximal ulna (arrows) and distal radius (arrowheads) are fractured. There is diffuse periosteal new bone surrounding the fracture sites (small arrows). (B) The lateral projection reveals an additional fracture of the distal humerus (open arrow).

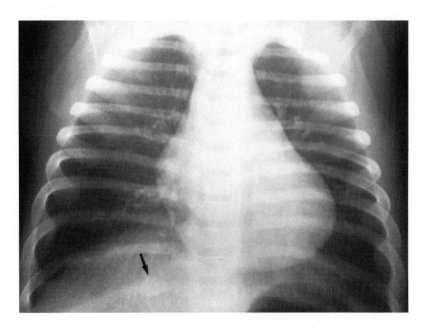

FIGURE 5-24 **AP chest radiograph: Healed rib fracture; child abuse:** The examination is normal with one exception; there is a healed posterior right rib fracture (arrow). This finding is subtle but led to a skeletal survey that revealed other healing fractures. This example of child abuse was not suspected clinically and illustrates the importance of careful radiographic observation.

normal position. The most frequently traumatized apophyseal centers are the medial epicondyle of the distal humerus (see Fig. 5-68), the lesser and greater trochanters, and the numerous growth centers of the juvenile pelvis (Figure 5-22).

Child Abuse

It is important that every child who comes to the emergency department because of trauma be evaluated for potential child abuse. Suspicion should in-crease if the trauma is greater than the clinical history suggests. Radiographically, a sure sign of child abuse is evidence of repeated injury. The diagnosis can be made if there are multiple fractures in various stages of healing (Figure 5-23). Rib fractures are almost always due to child abuse and can be difficult to detect (Figure 5-24). Other radiographic findings are either diagnostic or suggestive of abuse as indicated in Table 5-4. In children less than 1 year of age, metaphyseal fractures are the number-one fracture indicative of abuse. Metaphyseal bucket-handle or

TABLE 5-4 **Radiographic Indicators of Child Abuse**

Diagnostic of Abuse	Suspicious for Abuse
Metaphyseal corner fractures	Posterior rib fractures
Multiple fractures, various stages of healing	Fractures of the acromion, sternum, or spinous processes
Interhemispheric subdural hematoma	Fractures of the radius/ulna, tibia/fibula or femur in child less than 1 year of age
	Midshaft humeral fractures
	Any fracture more severe than expected by parental history
	Linear skull fractures
	Vertebral body fractures
	Subdural hematomas of varying age

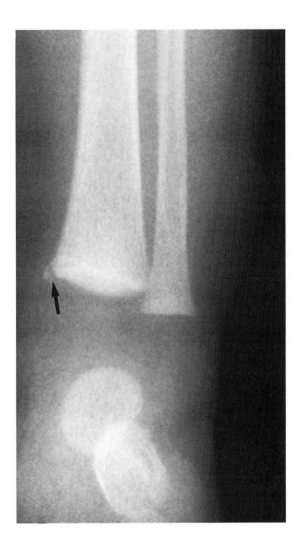

corner fractures are the hallmark of injury (Figure 5-25). Diaphyseal shaft fractures are the primary indicators of abuse in children older than 1 year of age. Evaluation of the potentially abused child is included in Algorithm 5-2.

ADULT ORTHOPEDIC TRAUMA

Upper Extremity Trauma

Shoulder   The glenohumeral joint is commonly dislocated. Glenohumeral dislocations are classified according to the relationship of the humeral head to the glenoid fossa. Anterior dislocations are the most common (Figure 5-26). Posterior dislocations are much less common and difficult to diagnose (Figure 5-27). Common complications of an anterior

←

FIGURE 5-25   **AP ankle: Metaphyseal corner fracture; child abuse:** There is a small metaphyseal corner fracture of this child's distal tibia (arrow). This finding is diagnostic of abuse and results from shaking the child violently by the extremity.

ALGORITHM 5-2   Evaluation of the Potentially Abused Child

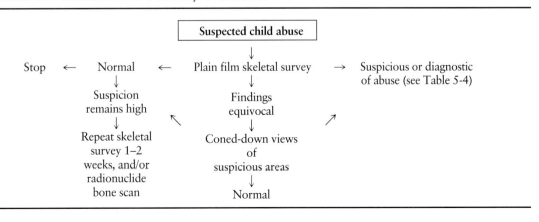

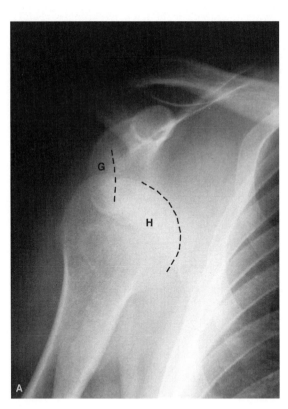
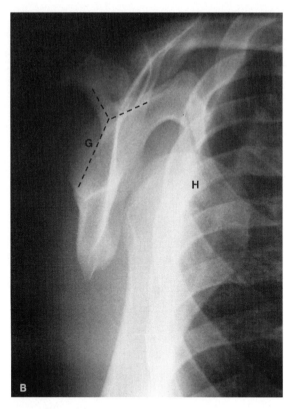

FIGURE 5-26 AP and "Y" views shoulder: Glenohumeral dislocation—Anterior: (A) AP view shows a dislocated humeral (H) head out of the glenoid (G) fossa. (B) The "Y" projection reveals anterior displacement of the humeral (H) head in relationship to the glenoid (G). No associated fracture is seen. However, anterior dislocations are associated with fractures of the greater tuberosity, glenoid rim, and humeral head. Postreduction views are necessary to exclude fracture.

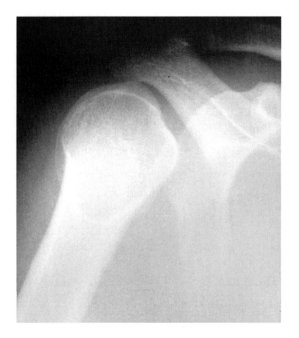

←

FIGURE 5-27 Single view shoulder: Glenohumeral dislocation—Posterior: The humeral head is fixed in internal rotation and there is widening of the shoulder joint. Both of these findings are characteristic of a posterior shoulder dislocation. Additional axillary or "Y" views should be obtained to confirm the diagnosis. Posterior dislocations are uncommon and are frequently caused by seizures. As in this case, radiographic findings are often subtle and frequently overlooked.

shoulder dislocation include a Hill-Sachs fracture of the humeral head, Bankart's fracture of the inferior glenoid, and fracture of the greater tuberosity (Figure 5-28). A Hill-Sachs fracture occurs when the dislocated humeral head impacts against the glenoid rim (Figure 5-29). Anterior dislocations can be complicated by rotator-cuff tears, especially in older individuals.

Clavicle Patients with clavicle fractures usually have a history of falling on an outstretched extremity. Most fractures occur in the middle third of the clavicle and are more common in children. Overriding of fracture fragments is a common finding (Figure 5-30). When the fracture involves the distal third of the clavicle, it is important to exclude injury to the distal clavicular ligaments and evaluate the integrity of the acromioclavicular joint.

Acromioclavicular (AC) Joint The normal AC joint is approximately 4 mm wide. The inferior clavicular cortical margin is aligned with the inferior margin of the acromion in most individuals (Figure 5-31). Trauma to the AC joint includes a spectrum of injuries from mild sprain to complete ligamentous disruption and AC dislocation (Figure 5-32). Radiographic examination of the AC joint requires special horizontal views. Additional stress images can be obtained by using weights to complete the evaluation.

Elbow The elbow is a complex joint consisting of three bony articulating surfaces. Evaluation of the elbow is centered not only around bony alignment but also on the elbow fat pads. The anterior fat pad is normally visualized in the anterior aspect of the

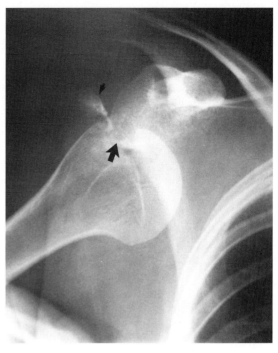

FIGURE 5-28 **AP view shoulder: Anterior dislocation with fracture of the greater tuberosity:** There is an anterior shoulder dislocation present complicated by a fracture of the greater tuberosity (large arrow). A small displaced fracture fragment is identified (small arrow).

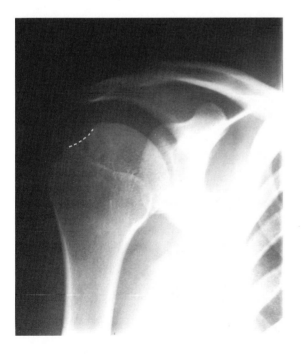

←

FIGURE 5-29 **AP shoulder: Hill-Sachs fracture:** AP view obtained after an anterior dislocation was reduced shows loss of the normal humeral head contour (dashed line). This Hill-Sachs fracture occurred as the dislocated humeral head impacted the glenoid. Most fractures occur posteriorly and are best seen on an internally rotated AP view.

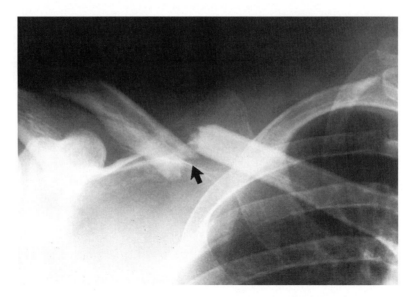

FIGURE 5-30   **AP clavicle: Fracture:** AP view shows a transverse fracture of the middle third of the clavicle (arrow). There is minimal overriding of the fracture fragments. The distal fragment is usually displaced caudally from the weight of the shoulder.

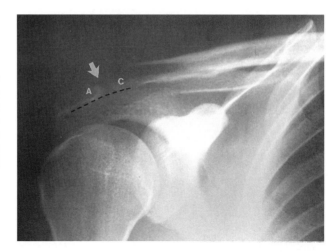

→

FIGURE 5-31   **AP view acromioclavicular joint: Normal:** The acromion (A) and distal clavicle (c) form the acromioclavicular joint (arrow). The inferior clavicular margin is normally aligned with the inferior acromion (dashed line). Evaluation of the acromioclavicular joint should include the width of the joint and position of the clavicle.

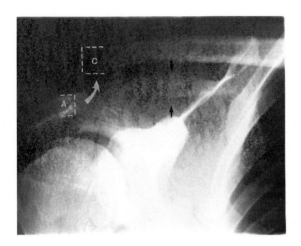

←

FIGURE 5-32   **AP view acromioclavicular (AC) joint: AC separation:** There is upward displacement of the distal clavicle (c) from the acromion (A) (curved arrow). The coracoclavicular space is increased representing disrupted ligaments (arrows). There is a spectrum of AC joint injury from mild strain through complete ligamentous disruption. Position of the clavicle in relation to the acromion, and coracoid process is essential to the diagnosis.

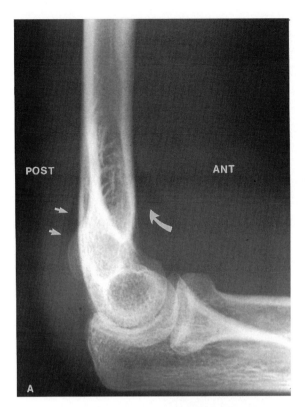
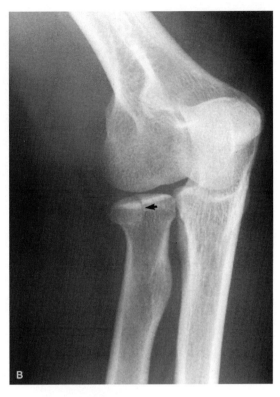

FIGURE 5-33   Oblique and lateral elbow radiographs: Hemarthrosis and radial head fracture: Close inspection of the traumatized elbow for a fat pad sign is extremely important. (A) This sign is detected on a true lateral projection by elevation of the anterior fat pad (curved arrow) and/or identifying a posterior fat pad (arrows). The fat pad sign is indicative of a hemarthrosis in the setting of trauma and is more commonly seen in pediatric patients. Fractures are present in up to 90% of children with a fat pad sign. No bony abnormality is seen on the lateral view. (B) The oblique view demonstrates a linear radial head fracture (arrow).

FIGURE 5-34   Normal anterior humeral and radiocapitellar lines: The anterior humeral line is drawn along the anterior humeral (H) cortex and extends through the capitellum (C) (large dashed line). This line normally passes through the middle third of the capitellum. The radiocapitellar line is drawn through the midradial (R) shaft and should normally pass through the capitellum (C) on any radiographic projection (small dashed line).

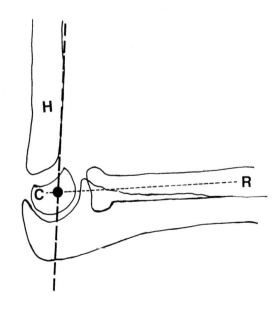

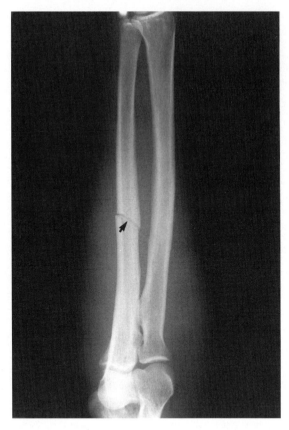

FIGURE 5-35   **PA forearm: Fractured ulna:** A fractured ulna is present (arrow) in this patient who was struck in the forearm by a baseball bat. It would be important to evaluate the lateral view for any fracture displacement and exclude dislocation of the proximal radius.

elbow on a lateral radiograph. The posterior fat pad is only seen when there is an intra-articular effusion that posteriorly displaces the fat out of its normal position in the intercondylar depression of the distal humerus. A fat pad sign refers to either elevation of the normal anterior fat pad that assumes a sail appearance or visualization of the posterior fat pad. These findings are diagnostic of a hemarthrosis in the setting of trauma. The posterior fat pad sign is usually a more sensitive indicator of joint fluid. In an adult, a radial head fracture is the most common cause of a hemarthrosis (Figure 5-33). Bony alignment is assessed by drawing the anterior hu-

meral line and the radiocapitellar line (Figure 5-34). These lines should normally pass through the mid-portion of the capitellum on any radiographic view. Failure to transect the capitellum is indicative of either a dislocated radial head or a displaced capitellum.

Forearm   Fractures of the distal radius and ulna are common. Most fractures of the forearm are easily recognized both clinically and radiographically. An isolated fracture of the ulna is termed a nightstick fracture and is usually the result of a direct blow to the forearm (Figure 5-35). A Monteggia fracture consists of a fracture of the proximal third of the ulna

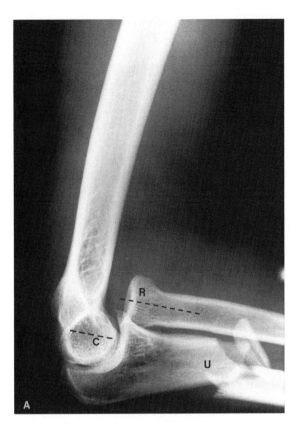

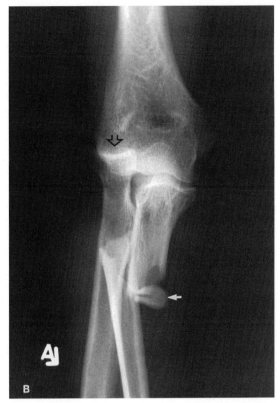

FIGURE 5-36 **AP and lateral elbow: Monteggia's fracture:** (A) Lateral projection demonstrates the typical Monteggia's fracture consisting of a proximal ulna (u) fracture with an associated dislocated radial (R) head. An important diagnostic key is that a line drawn through the long axis of the radius should intersect the capitellum (C) on any view. In this case, the radial head is dislocated anteriorly (dashed line). (B) The AP view shows the comminuted ulnar fracture (arrow) with radial displacement of the distal fragment. There is a double density over the lateral epicondyle representing the dislocated radial head (open arrow).

with associated dislocation of the proximal radius (Figure 5-36). The radiocapitellar line will be disrupted. A Galeazzi fracture is a fracture of the mid to distal third of the radius in association with dislocation of the radial ulnar joint. These injuries stress the importance of radiographically evaluating the joints above and below fractures for any abnormality. A Colles' fracture results from falling on an outstretched hand and consists of a comminuted fracture of the distal radius with dorsal angulation at the fracture site (Figure 5-37). This assumes a characteristic "silver-fork" deformity. Radial head fractures are associated with Colles' fractures.

Wrist Evaluating the wrist can be difficult due to the number of carpal bones and their relationship with one another. The normal wrist consists of two rows with four carpal bones in each row (Figure 5-38). When evaluating the wrist, it is important to inspect the integrity of all cortical surfaces and the position of each carpal bone. Close inspection of the carpal articulations, especially the lunate and capitate is important when evaluating the wrist for possible carpal dislocation or subluxation. Ligamentous injury is a common sequela of wrist trauma. Rotary subluxation of the scaphoid or scapholunate disassociation occurs with acute dorsiflexion of the wrist,

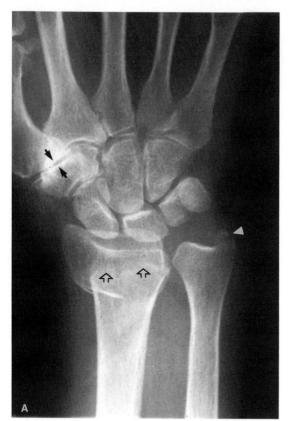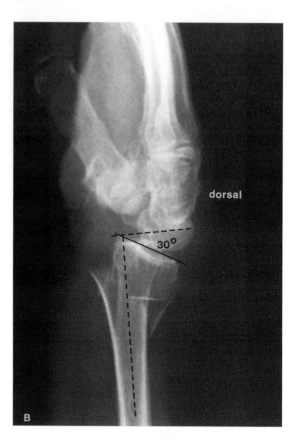

FIGURE 5-37   PA and lateral wrist: Colles' fracture: (A) PA view shows a transverse fracture of the distal radius (open arrows) and ulnar styloid (arrowhead). Degenerative disease is present at the base of the thumb (arrows). (B) Lateral projection reveals 30 degrees of dorsal angulation of the radial articular surface. This measurement is calculated by drawing a line through the long axis of the radial shaft and a second line perpendicular to the first (dashed lines). The angle of inclination is then calculated by drawing a third line along the radial articular surface (solid line). A normal wrist has approximately 10 degrees of volar tilt.

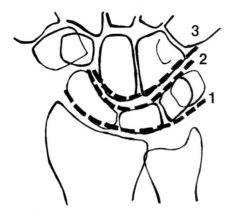

Normal Carpal Arcs

FIGURE 5-38   Normal carpal arcs: Joining the articular margins of the two rows of carpal bones should form these smooth parallel arcs. Any disruption of these arcs is abnormal and usually indicates a malpositioned carpal bone(s).

$\rightarrow$

FIGURE 5-39 **PA wrist: Scapholunate dissociation:** There is an abnormally widened space (arrow) between the scaphoid (S) and lunate (L). This occurs secondary to tearing of numerous interosseous ligaments with rotary subluxation of the scaphoid. There is an association between scapholunate dissociation and fractures of the distal radius.

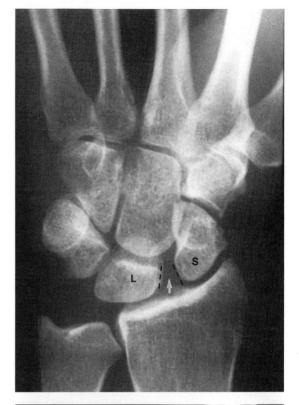

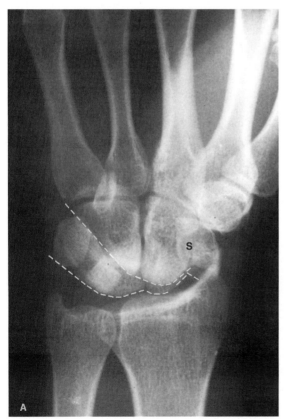

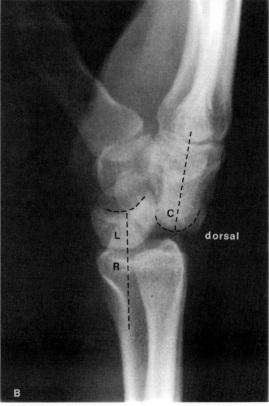

FIGURE 5-40 **PA and lateral wrist: Perilunate dislocation with scaphoid fracture:** (A) The PA view reveals disrupted carpal arcs as well as a fractured scaphoid (S). (B) The lateral projection shows dorsal dislocation of the capitate (C). The lunate (L) maintains a normal relationship with the radius (R). Most perilunate dislocations result from falling on an outstretched hand and are associated with scaphoid fractures.

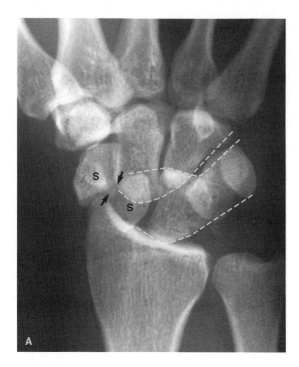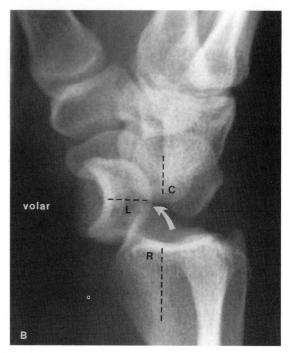

FIGURE 5-41   **PA and lateral wrist: Lunate dislocation with scaphoid fracture:** (A) PA view shows abnormal carpal arcs. The scaphoid (S) is fractured into two displaced pieces (arrows). (B) The lateral view demonstrates volar displacement of the lunate (L) disrupting the normal capitate (C), lunate (L) and radial (R) alignment (curved arrow).

which tears the interosseous ligaments of the lunate, scaphoid, and capitate bones. This ligamentous disruption results in a widening between the scaphoid bone. A distance of ≥4 mm is probably abnormal (Figure 5-39). A perilunate dislocation may be somewhat confusing in its appearance; however, careful inspection of the carpal relationship on lateral view will demonstrate an abnormal capitate, lunate, and radial alignment. The distal carpal row is most commonly dislocated dorsally. The lunate maintains its normal alignment with the radius (Figure 5-40). A lunate dislocation is demonstrated by a volar displacement of the lunate with disruption of the normal carpal alignment (Figure 5-41). Most carpal dislocations are associated with carpal fractures. These fractures may be difficult to identify due to the disrupted carpal arcs and unusual carpal bone alignment. In summary, when confronted with a confusing carpal bone appearance, pay close attention to the alignment of the radius, lunate, and capitate.

A scaphoid fracture is commonly caused by falling on an outstretched hand. The patient feels pain in the anatomic snuffbox. A nondisplaced transverse fracture of the midportion or waist of the scaphoid bone is the most common (Figure 5-42). Most scaphoid fractures are isolated injuries; however, they can be seen in combination with both Colles' fractures of the forearm and radial head fractures. Due to the unusual blood supply of the scaphoid bone, scaphoid fractures have a high incidence of nonunion and avascular necrosis of the proximal fragment. It is extremely important to establish the diagnosis early and initiate therapy to avoid complications. In the appropriate clinical setting and with negative radiographs, special scaphoid views or a radionuclide bone scan may be necessary for proper evaluation. Triquetral fractures are usually small avulsion fractures that are characteristically seen only on the lateral view of the wrist. Soft-tissue swelling is seen in association with the fracture (Figure 5-43).

Hand   Fractures of the metacarpals and phalanges are common. The boxer's fracture is a characteristic metacarpal injury involving a transverse fracture of the distal fourth or fifth metacarpal. Dorsal apex angulation at the fracture site is common (Figure 5-44). These patients have a history of striking a blow with a clenched fist.

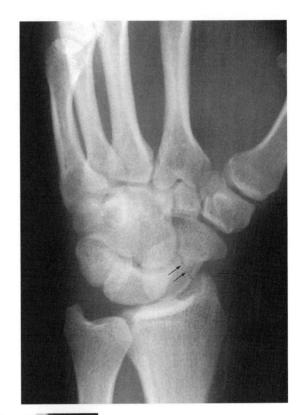

$\rightarrow$

FIGURE 5-42 PA wrist: Scaphoid fracture: There is a nondisplaced transverse fracture of the waist of the scaphoid (arrows).

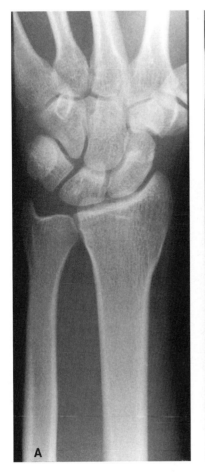

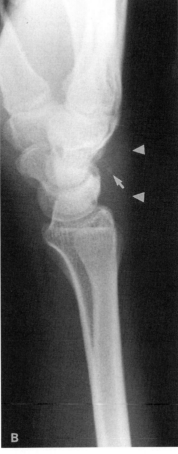

FIGURE 5-43 PA and lateral wrist: Triquetral fracture: (A) The PA view is normal. (B) The lateral projection shows a small triquetral avulsion fracture (arrow) with soft-tissue swelling (arrowheads).

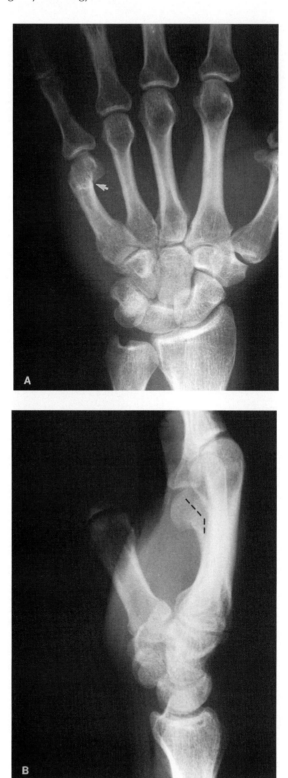

FIGURE 5-44 PA and lateral hand: Boxer's fracture: (A) The PA view reveals a fracture of the distal fifth metacarpal (arrow). (B) The lateral projection demonstrates characteristic dorsal apex angulation at the fracture site (dashed lines).

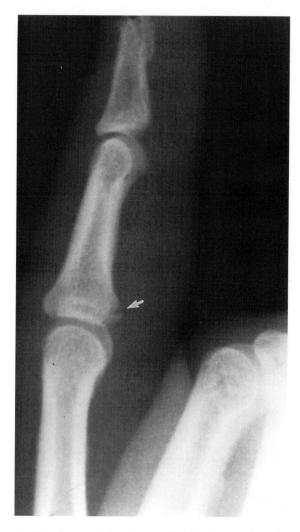

FIGURE 5-45   **Lateral finger: Avulsion fracture:** There is a small volar plate avulsion fracture at the base of the middle phalanx (arrow). This fracture is usually the result of a hyperextension injury.

Avulsion fractures of the fingers are common and occur at tendinous insertions (Figure 5-45). Due to their small size, these fractures can be difficult to detect on plain films. Oblique views are often helpful in making the diagnosis.

Dislocation of a digit occurs frequently and is usually the result of hyperextension forces. Dorsal dislocations are the most common (Figure 5-46). It is important to obtain postreduction radiographs to exclude an associated fracture.

Special radiographic views are required to evaluate the injured thumb. Fractures of the base of the thumb may be either intra- or extra-articular. A Bennett's fracture consists of a fracture-dislocation at the base of the first metacarpal (Figure 5-47).

Pelvis   The pelvis is a ring structure composed of two arches. The posterior arch is a major weight-bearing arch composed of the iliac wings and sacrum that extends posteriorly and superiorly from the acetabula. The anterior arch extends inferior and anterior from the acetabula. It is important to know, clinically, that isolated fractures through the pelvic ring are uncommon. When encountering what appears to be an isolated pelvic fracture, careful inspection of all cortical surfaces and the sacroiliac (SI) joints should be made. Diastasis of one or both SI joints occurs frequently with pelvic fractures (Figure 5-48). The degree of diastasis can be subtle, and CT may be necessary for proper evaluation. It is also important to inspect the sacral arcuate lines to exclude fracture. A single break in the pelvic ring, such as an isolated pubic ramus fracture, is stable. Most stable pelvic fractures involve the anterior arch and represent the majority of pelvic trauma. Unstable

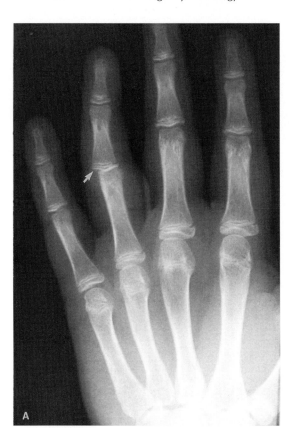

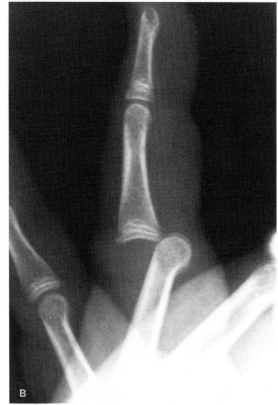

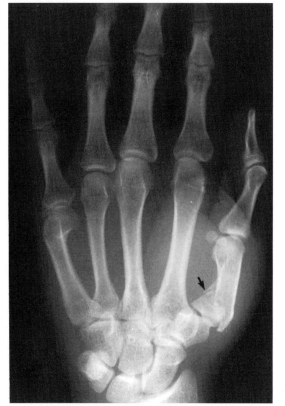

FIGURE 5-46   **PA hand and lateral fourth finger: Dorsal dislocation:** (A) PA view demonstrates an abnormal fourth proximal interphalangeal joint (arrow). (B) The lateral view shows dorsal dislocation of the digit. Dorsal dislocations are the most common type of dislocation. Radiographs need to be closely scrutinized for any associated fracture, particularly of the volar plate.

←

FIGURE 5-47   **PA hand: Bennett's fracture base of the thumb:** There is an oblique fracture of the base of the thumb (arrow) with lateral dislocation of the first metacarpal. This fracture-dislocation complex is referred to as a Bennett's fracture.

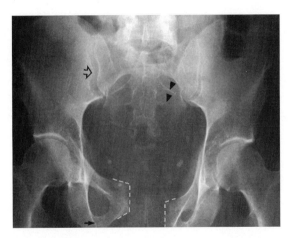

FIGURE 5-48 **AP pelvis: Pelvic fracture:** This patient presented after an automobile accident. There is diastasis of both the pubic symphysis (dashed lines) as well as the right sacroiliac joint (open arrow). A nondisplaced fracture of the inferior right pubic ramus is also seen (arrow). It is important to carefully inspect the sacral arcuate lines for any fractures. In this case they are normal (arrowheads).

pelvic fractures are the result of multiple fractures usually involving both the anterior and posterior arches. Unstable pelvic fractures are the result of severe trauma and are associated with head, chest, abdominal, and orthopedic injuries. Types of unstable pelvic fractures are represented in Figure 5-49. Pelvic fractures are associated with severe and sometimes life-threatening hemorrhage, as well as genitourinary tract injuries. Additional plain film views,

such as inlet/outlet or Judet views may help to further characterize pelvic fractures. CT plays a significant role in the evaluation of pelvic trauma. CT superbly evaluates the acetabula and SI joints and demonstrates displacement of fracture fragments (Figure 5-50). An additional benefit of CT is the ability to evaluate adjacent soft tissues for hematoma or bladder disruption.

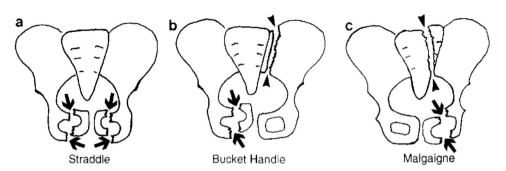

FIGURE 5-49 **Types of unstable pelvic fractures:** (a) Straddle pelvic fracture consists of fractures through all four pubic rami (arrows). The fracture fragments are usually displaced cephalad. Straddle fractures are associated with both bladder and urethral injuries. (b) Bucket-handle pelvic fracture is a type of double-vertical fracture. Both anterior and posterior arches are disrupted. However, the fractures are on opposite sides. This illustration demonstrates fractures through the pubic rami (arrows) in association with contralateral disruption of the sacroiliac joint (arrowheads). (c) Malgaigne pelvic fracture is a double-vertical fracture through ipsilateral anterior and posterior pelvic arches. This illustration demonstrates fractured pubic rami (arrows) with an associated sacral fracture (arrowheads).

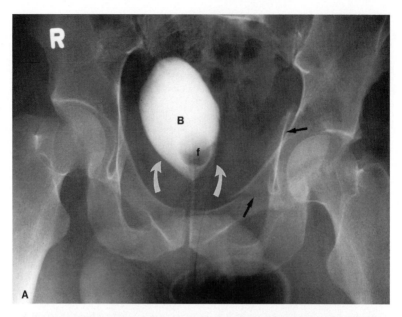

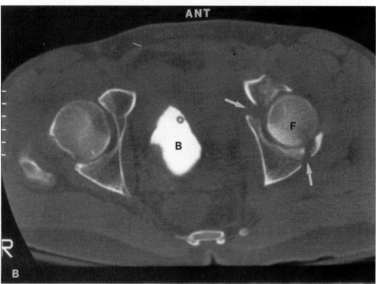

FIGURE 5-50   **AP radiograph and CT pelvis: Fracture left acetabulum:** (A) AP pelvis shows a fracture of the left acetabulum (arrows). A cystogram was performed by instilling iodinated contrast into the patient's bladder (B) through the Foley catheter (f). The bladder is deformed and elevated by a pelvic hematoma (curved arrows). (B) Axial CT filmed with bone technique demonstrates fractures through the anterior and posterior columns of the left acetabulum (arrows). The femoral head (F) is normally located in the acetabulum. Contrast in the bladder is again seen.

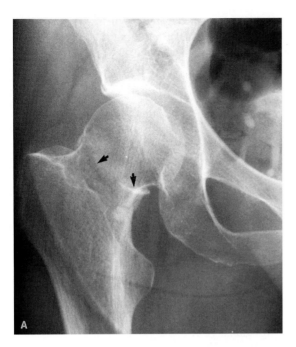
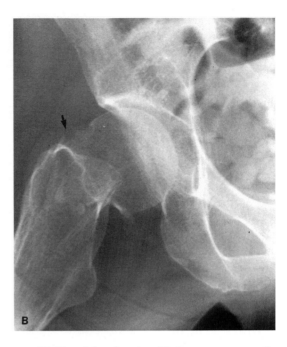

FIGURE 5-51 **AP and frog-leg views hip: Subcapital hip fracture:** AP (A) and frog-leg view (B) demonstrate a nondisplaced subcapital hip fracture (arrows). Subcapital fractures occur at the junction of the femoral head and neck and are the most common type of hip fracture.

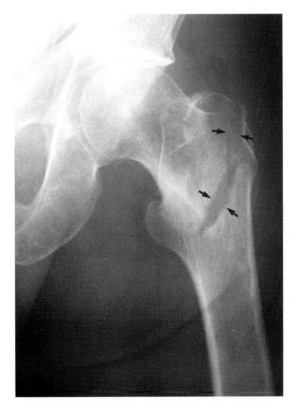

FIGURE 5-52 **AP hip: Intertrochanteric hip fracture:** A diagonal fracture line is seen extending from the greater to the lesser trochanter (arrows).

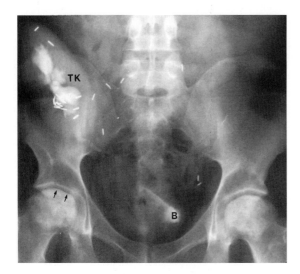

← FIGURE 5-53 **AP pelvis: Bilateral avascular necrosis (AVN) of the femoral heads:** Single view of the pelvis was performed as part of an intravenous urogram. The patient has a transplanted kidney (TK) in the right iliac fossa. Contrast is seen in the collecting system as well as the patient's bladder (B). The femoral heads are sclerotic, and there is irregularity of the joint surface (arrows). This case of bilateral AVN was due to chronic steroid usage.

Hip Hip fractures are considered synonymous with "old age" due to age-related osteoporosis. Plain films are usually sufficient to diagnose a hip fracture. There are instances, however, in which the patient is symptomatic and plain films are essentially normal. Radionuclide bone scanning or MRI may be of benefit in detecting radiographically occult fractures in these patients. Generally, hip fractures are classified as subcapital (Figure 5-51), femoral neck, intratrochanteric (Figure 5-52), and subtrochanteric.

Avascular necrosis of the hip has numerous etiologies. Trauma, alcoholism, steroid usage, pancreatitis, and vasculitis are common causes. The patient usually has hip pain. Radiographic detection may be difficult in the early stages, but as the disease progresses, a characteristic subcortical fracture occurs. Progression of the disease results in deformity and sclerosis of the femoral head (Figure 5-53). Early diagnosis of suspected AVN can sometimes be made with MRI.

Traumatic hip dislocations usually occur posteriorly and are commonly the sequela of motor vehicle accidents (Figure 5-54). Following hip relocation, CT plays a valuable role in visualizing the hip joint to exclude any entrapped bone fragments, femoral head fractures, or acetabular fractures. The posterior acetabulum is the most common fracture associated with posterior hip dislocations.

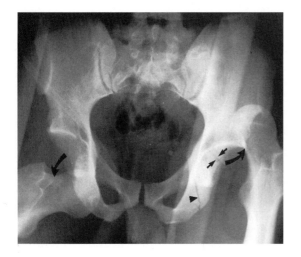

← FIGURE 5-54 **AP pelvis: Bilateral hip dislocations with fractures:** Both hips are dislocated (curved arrows). Nondisplaced fractures are detected in the left ischium (arrowhead) and left acetabulum (arrows). Posterior dislocations are more common than anterior dislocations and have a higher incidence of complications. Complications of posterior dislocations include avascular necrosis of the femoral head and early degenerative joint disease.

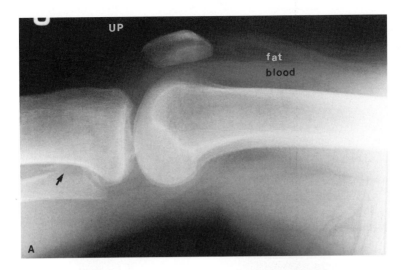

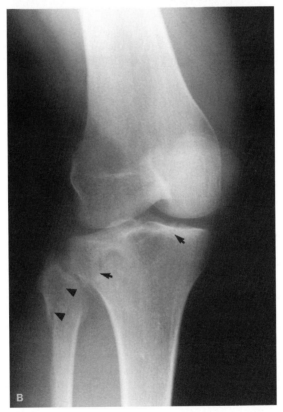

FIGURE 5-55   Oblique and cross-table knee radiographs: Lateral tibial plateau fracture: (A) Cross-table (horizontal beam) radiograph shows a lipohemarthrosis (fat-blood) level in the suprapatellar bursa. A minimally displaced fracture of the proximal fibula is present (arrow). (B) The oblique view demonstrates a minimally depressed lateral tibial plateau fracture (arrows). The fibular fracture is again seen (arrowheads). Most tibial plateau fractures occur after a twisting injury and commonly involve the lateral tibial plateau. A lipohemarthrosis is highly suggestive of an intra-articular fracture but its absence does not exclude such an injury.

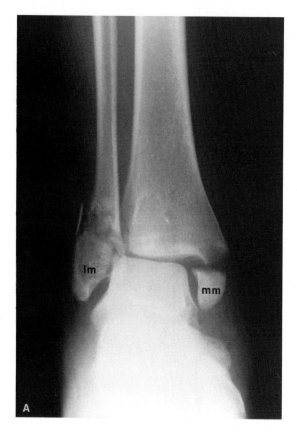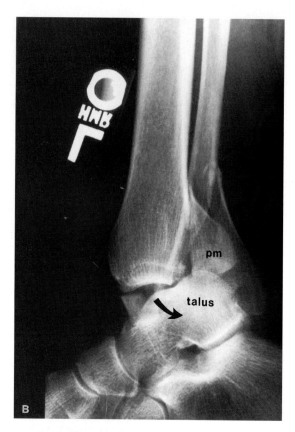

FIGURE 5-56   **AP and lateral ankle: Trimalleolar fracture-dislocation:** (A) AP view shows fractures of both the medial malleolus (mm) and lateral malleolus (lm). The talus and medial malleolus are displaced laterally. (B) The lateral view demonstrates a fracture of the posterior malleolus (pm) as well as posterior dislocation of the talus (curved arrow).

Knee   Patients presenting with knee trauma usually have normal radiographs. It is important to obtain a cross-table or horizontal-beam radiograph to examine for a lipohemarthrosis. A lipohemarthrosis is identified by a fat-blood level, usually in the region of the suprapatellar bursa. This is indicative of an intra-articular fracture, usually a fracture of the lateral tibial plateau (Figure 5-55). In the absence of a fracture, a hemarthrosis may indicate intra-articular soft-tissue derangement, particularly a torn anterior cruciate ligament. There is a spectrum of tibial plateau fractures from mild bony depression through comminuted fractures. Mild depressions may be difficult to detect, and CT with multiplanar image reconstruction may be necessary to identify the degree of fracture fragment depression.

Knee dislocations are rare but they are true orthopedic emergencies. Vascular damage, which frequently accompanies the dislocation, requires emergent diagnosis and treatment if the extremity is to be saved.

Ankle   The ankle is a complex joint composed of the tibia, fibula, and talus, as well as numerous ligamentous structures. It is the most frequently injured joint of the body. Radiographic manifestations of trauma to the ankle joint include not only bony fractures but ligamentous injury that can be difficult to detect in the acute setting. Widening of the ankle mortise, overlying soft-tissue swelling, as well as evidence for a joint effusion are indicators of soft-tissue injury. The majority of ankle trauma consists of inversion injuries with sprains of the lateral collateral ligaments. Stress views may be necessary to exclude significant soft tissue damage. Bony fractures include isolated malleolar fractures, bimalleolar fractures, or tri-malleolar fractures. A tri-malleolar fracture consists of fractures through both the lateral and medial malleoli seen in conjunction with a posterior tibial lip fracture (Figure 5-56). These are commonly associated with dislocations. Isolated posterior tibial lip and nondisplaced

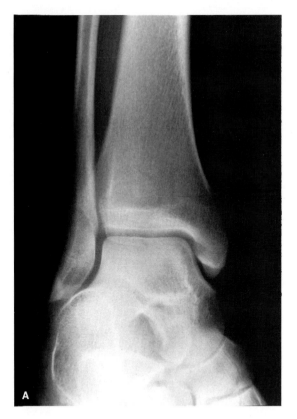 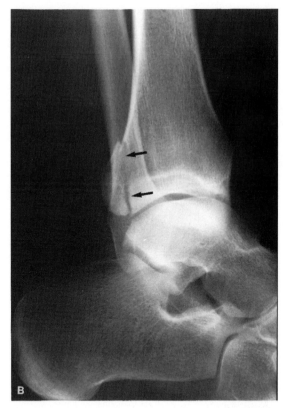

FIGURE 5-57 Oblique and lateral view ankle: Posterior tibial lip or posterior malleolus fracture: (A) The oblique view is normal. (B) Lateral projection shows an isolated posterior tibial lip fracture. These injuries are associated with Maissoneuve's fractures of the proximal fibula. This is another example of how important multiple projections are in diagnosing skeletal trauma.

oblique distal fibular fractures are sometimes seen only on the lateral view (Figure 5-57).

A Maisonneuve fracture is a fracture of the proximal shaft of the fibula in association with injury or fracture of the ankle (Figure 5-58). It is important to examine the lower extremity to exclude proximal fibular trauma in patients who have ankle injuries.

Foot Radiographic interpretation of foot films can be difficult due to the presence of numerous secondary or accessory centers of ossification. Additional diagnostic difficulty can be encountered with pediatric foot radiographs due to growth centers. A common source of error in this regard is misinterpreting the apophysis at the base of the fifth metatarsal for a fracture (Figure 5-59).

The calcaneus is the most frequently fractured tarsal bone (Figure 5-60). Calculation of Boehler's angle is useful when evaluating the calcaneus for

potential fracture (Figure 5-61). A normal Boehler's angle measures between 20 and 40 degrees. Less than 20 degrees should raise suspicion for calcaneal fracture. There is a well known association of calcaneal fractures with spinal fractures and contralateral foot and ankle injuries.

A Lisfranc fracture-dislocation occurs through the tarsal metatarsal joints (Figure 5-62). These fracture-dislocations occur commonly in young children and neuropathic joints. Radiographic findings may be subtle and misdiagnosis is common. It is important to ensure that the lateral aspect of the first metatarsal is appropriately aligned with the medial cuneiform bone and that the medial border of the second metatarsal is aligned with the medial border of the middle cuneiform.

Fractures through the base of the fifth metatarsal are transverse in orientation, distinguishing them from the apophysis (Figure 5-63).

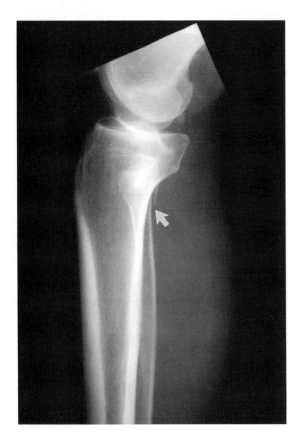

←

FIGURE 5-58 **Lateral view tibia-fibula: Maisonneuve fracture:** A minimally displaced fracture of the proximal fibula is visible (arrow) in a patient with ankle trauma. Radiographs of the ankle were normal. However, there was palpable tenderness in the lateral knee. This represents a Maisonneuve fracture and illustrates the importance of a complete physical examination of the injured extremity.

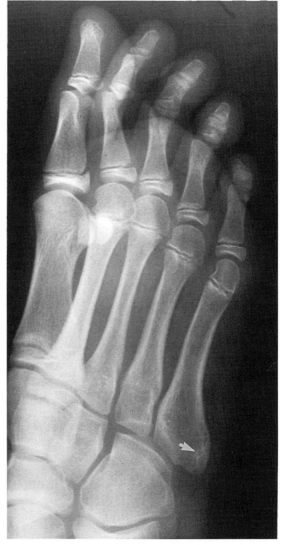

→

FIGURE 5-59 **Oblique foot: Normal apophysis:** The apophysis at the base of the fifth metatarsal is aligned parallel to the metatarsal shaft (arrow). This should not be mistaken for a fracture. Fractures are oriented in a transverse plane (see Figure 5-63).

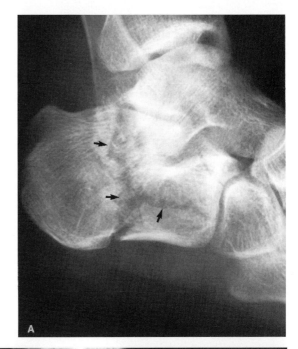

FIGURE 5-60   Multiple lateral calcaneal radiographs:
Various fractures: (A) Multiple fracture lines are present
in this comminuted calcaneal fracture (arrows). This type
of injury usually occurs after the patient jumps or falls
from a high place and then lands on their feet. Boehler's
angle is abnormal. (B) A nondisplaced linear fracture of
the calcaneus is present (arrows). Boehler's angle is normal. (C) Lateral projection shows a minimally displaced
fracture of the anterior calcaneus. Boehler's angle is abnormal.

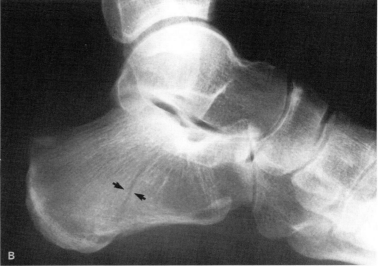

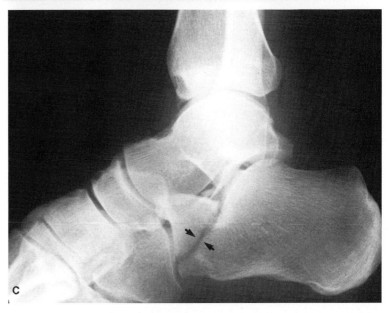

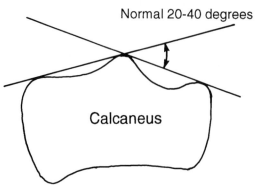

FIGURE 5-61 Boehler's Angle: Boehler's angle is calculated on lateral foot digraphs by drawing intersecting lines as illustrated above. The normal Boehler's angle measures 20 to 40 degrees. Abnormal measurements are highly suspicious for calcaneal fracture.

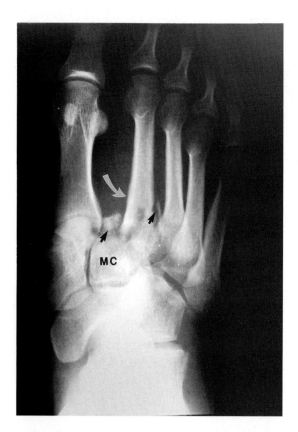

FIGURE 5-62 AP foot radiograph: Lisfranc fracture-dislocation: Lateral dislocation of the second through fifth tarsometatarsal joints is present (curved arrow). Avulsion fractures are seen at the base of the second metatarsal (arrows). It is important to notice the second metatarsal is misaligned with the middle cuneiform (mc) bone to detect the dislocation. Comparison views may assist in the diagnosis.

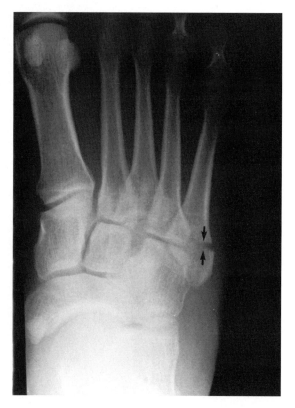

FIGURE 5-63 AP foot radiograph: Fractured fifth metatarsal: There is a minimally displaced transverse fracture at the base of the fifth metatarsal (arrows). This avulsion fracture results from forceful inversion of the foot.

PLAIN FILM DETECTION OF SOFT-TISSUE ABNORMALITIES

It is frequently possible to localize or confirm the presence of a soft-tissue, radiopaque, foreign body with plain films. Plain film technique may need to be altered, depending on the composition of the suspected foreign body. Metal and certain types of glass are usually well imaged (Figure 5-64). Wood products, however, are rarely seen. If the foreign body can be seen on plain films, then fluoroscopy can be used to assist in its removal. Air within the soft tissues may be due to infection (Figure 5-65), skin laceration, or pulmonary air leaks, i.e., subcutaneous air from a pneumothorax (Figure 3-68). Air in joints or vertebral disc spaces is due to chronic degenerative disease, and its presence virtually excludes infection.

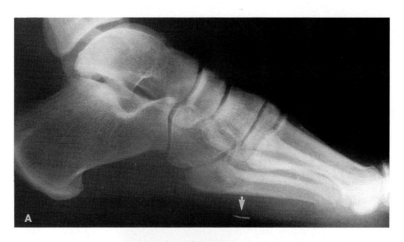

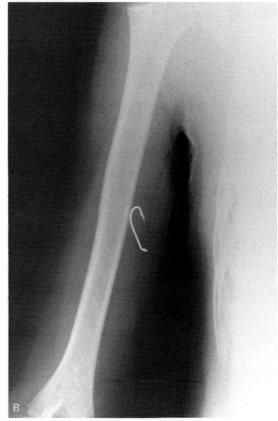

FIGURE 5-64 **Lateral foot and AP humerus: Soft-tissue foreign bodies:** (A) Lateral foot film was obtained in this young woman after she stepped on a sewing needle. The needle fragments are easily seen in the superficial tissues of the foot (arrows). (B) A fish hook is easily identified in the medial aspect of this child's arm. This film was obtained because the hook was completely imbedded in the soft tissues, and there was concern for possible neurovascular injury.

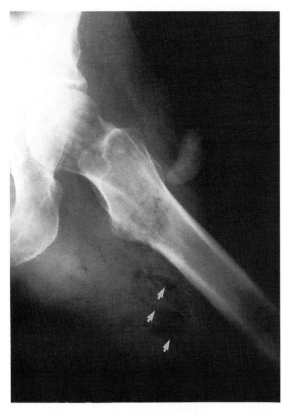

FIGURE 5-65 **Frog-leg lateral hip: Necrotizing fascitis:** Linear pockets of air are seen throughout the soft tissues of the thigh (arrows). This is an ominous finding representing a severe and life threatening infection. This patient died from overwhelming sepsis 12 hours after this film.

difficult to detect. Evaluation of the true lateral radiograph is of the utmost importance. Inspection of both the fat pads for displacement or elevation, as well as the anterior humeral line, will be necessary to accurately make the diagnosis.

Avulsion of the medial epicondyle can occur with a hard throwing motion and has been termed "Little Leaguer's Elbow" (Figure 5-68).

Lifting a child by the arm can result in subluxing the nonossified radial head under the annular ligament. This is known as a nursemaid's elbow. Plain films are rarely useful as they will appear normal. Manipulating the forearm usually unlocks the radial head from the annular ligament and quickly relieves the child's discomfort.

Hip

Legg-Perthes disease is an idiopathic avascular necrosis of the proximal femoral epiphysis occurring during childhood. Radiographic appearance of the hip depends on the stage of the disease. Initial radiographs may be normal; however, as the disease progresses, the proximal femoral epiphysis will become sclerotic and irregular in its appearance (Figure 5-69).

An overweight adolescent presenting with hip pain and a limp is suggestive of a slipped capital femoral epiphysis (SCFE). Most cases are idiopathic, although it is postulated that it may be hormonally

PEDIATRIC ORTHOPEDIC PROBLEMS

Clavicle

As in adults, clavicle fractures occur commonly after falling on an extended arm (Figure 5-66). Diagnosis may be difficult if the fracture is a green-stick or a bowing type injury. In this regard, contralateral radiographs or an apical lordotic view may be beneficial.

Elbow

In the pediatric patient, there are numerous ossification centers that can cause difficulty in radiographic interpretation. A textbook of normal variants as well as contralateral radiographs are beneficial for difficult cases. The most common fracture involving the pediatric elbow joint is the supracondylar fracture of the distal humerus (Figure 5-67). This injury usually results from falling on an outstretched extremity. Most injuries are clearly visible; however, subtle nondisplaced fractures may be

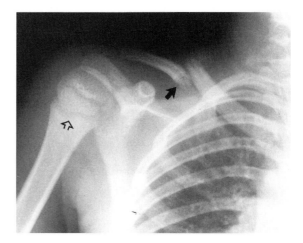

FIGURE 5-66 **AP shoulder: Clavicle fracture:** An easily identifiable clavicle fracture is seen in this child (arrow). However, many pediatric clavicle fractures are green-stick or bow type injuries. In these instances, the diagnosis can be difficult and may require apical lordotic or contralateral clavicle films for the diagnosis. The proximal humeral physis should not be mistaken for a fracture (open arrow).

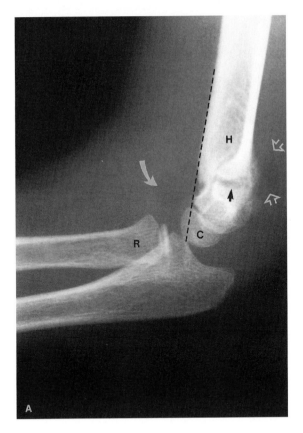

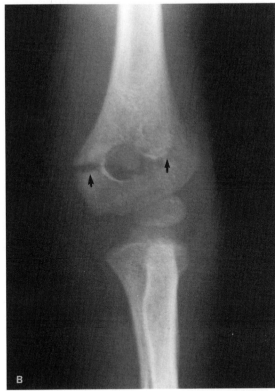

FIGURE 5-67 **AP and lateral elbow: Supracondylar fracture distal humerus:** (A) The lateral projection demonstrates a hemarthrosis as there is elevation of the anterior fat pad (curved arrow) and displacement of the posterior fat pad (open arrows). A fracture through the supracondylar humerus (H) is present (arrow). The radius (R) is normally aligned with the capitellum (C). However, there is posterior displacement of the distal humeral fragment as the anterior humeral line (dashed line) is abnormal. It should pass through the middle third of the capitellum, but in this case it passes through the anterior third. (B) AP view clearly shows a transverse fracture through the distal humerus (arrows).

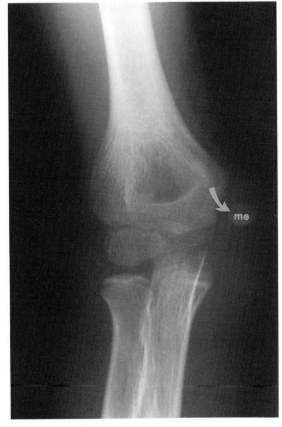

$\rightarrow$

FIGURE 5-68 **AP view elbow: Little Leaguer's elbow:** The medial epicondyle (me) is avulsed and displaced inferiorly (curved arrow). This is an example of a Salter-Harris I fracture.

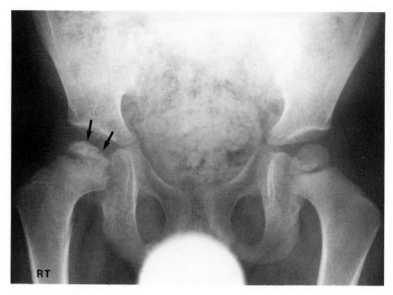

FIGURE 5-69   AP pelvis: Legg-Perthes disease: The right proximal femoral epiphysis is small, sclerotic, and has an irregular epiphyseal margin (arrows). These findings represent advanced Legg-Perthes disease. This patient had presented to the emergency department 2 months prior with an acute limp. Initial radiographs were interpreted as normal. The patient was lost to follow-up until he returned with a history of chronic right hip pain.

related. Plain films demonstrate widening and irregularity of the proximal femoral physis with medial displacement of the epiphysis. On AP hip radiographs, a line drawn along the outer aspect of the femoral neck should intersect the normal femoral capital epiphysis, but will miss the SCFE. A SCFE may best be detected by frog-leg views of the hips to visualize the medial displaced epiphysis (Figure 5-70).

Lower Extremity

A toddler's fracture has classically been described as a spiral fracture of the distal tibia (Figure 5-71). A child with this fracture usually has a limp or is unwilling to bear weight on the affected extremity. The important clinical point is to distinguish these characteristic fractures from fractures related to child abuse.

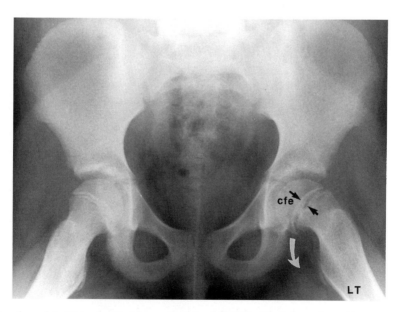

FIGURE 5-70   Frog-leg pelvis: Slipped capital femoral epiphysis (SCFE): The left epiphyseal line is widened (arrows) and the femoral head has slipped medially (curved arrow). The frog-leg projection is an extremely important view to obtain when there is clinical concern for a SCFE.

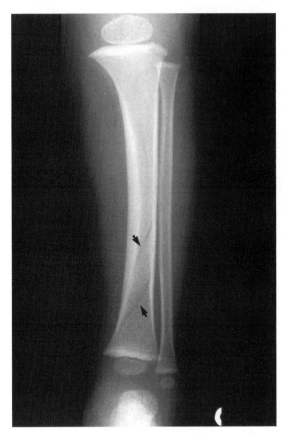

FIGURE 5-71 AP tibia-fibula: Toddler's fracture: A nondisplaced oblique tibial fracture is present (arrows). This is the characteristic finding of a toddler's fracture. Toddler's fractures are most common in children between 1 and 3 years old. The child usually presents with a limp.

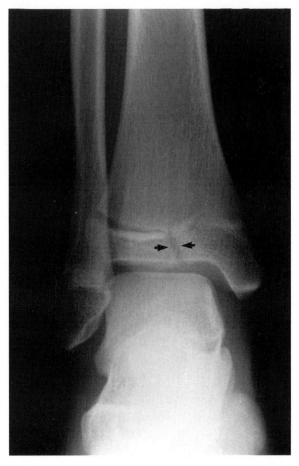

FIGURE 5-72 AP ankle: Fracture distal tibial epiphysis: There is a vertical fracture through the distal tibial epiphysis (arrows). This represents a Salter-Harris III injury and is also known as a Juvenile Tillaux fracture.

Ankle fractures in the juvenile population usually involve the epiphysis (Figure 5-72). This is because ligamentous structures in children are stronger than their growth plates.

Chapter 5 Orthopedic Pearls

1. Radiograph areas of suspected bony trauma in a minimum of two perpendicular views.
2. Radiograph joints above and below fractures to exclude subluxations or dislocations.
3. Avulsion fractures of the pelvis are common in young and adolescent patients.
4. Always exclude child abuse in cases of pediatric trauma.
5. The inability to externally rotate the shoulder is a classic finding with a posterior shoulder dislocation.
6. Pay careful attention to elbow fat pads to detect a hemarthrosis.
7. A fat/blood level (lipohemarthrosis) on horizontal beam X-ray is virtually diagnostic of an intra-articular fracture. This is an especially useful view to obtain following knee trauma.
8. Scaphoid fractures can be radiographically occult. Special scaphoid views with ulnar deviation of the hand may be useful.
9. A limping child who cannot localize the area of pain should have radiographs of the pelvis, femur, tibia-fibula, foot, and possibly the lumbar spine.
10. Many ankle injuries are associated with fractures of the proximal fibula. Be sure to examine the entire lower extremity.
11. Always exclude a fracture of the base of the fifth metatarsal on lateral ankle radiographs. Pain may be referred from the foot to the ankle, causing some diagnostic confusion.

Suggested Readings

1. Harris JH Jr, Edeiken-Monroe B. The Radiology of Acute Cervical Spine Trauma. 2nd ed. Baltimore: Williams & Wilkins; 1987.
2. Harris JH Jr, Harris WH, Novelline RA. The Radiology of Emergency Medicine. 3rd ed. Baltimore: Williams & Wilkins; 1993.
3. Keats TE. Emergency Radiology. 2nd ed. Chicago: Year Book Medical Publishers; 1989.
4. Keats TE. An Atlas of Normal Roentgen Variants that may Simulate Disease. 3rd ed. Chicago: Year Book Medical Publishers; 1984.
5. Redman HC, Miller GL, Purdy PD, Rollins NK. Emergency Radiology. Philadelphia: WB Saunders; 1993.
6. Rogers LF, Hendrix RW. Radiology of Skeletal Trauma. vols. 1 & 2. 2nd ed. New York: Churchill Livingstone; 1992.
7. Rosen P, Doris PE, Barkin RM, Barkin SZ, Markovchick VJ, eds. Diagnostic Radiology in Emergency Medicine. St. Louis; Mosby Year Book; 1992.
8. Swischuk LE. Emergency Imaging of the Acutely Ill or Injured Child. 3rd ed. Baltimore: Williams & Wilkins; 1994.
9. Weissman BNW, Sledge CG. Orthopedic Radiology. Philadelphia: WB Saunders Company; 1986.

Index

Note: Page numbers in *italics* refer to illustrations; page numbers followed by t refer to tables.